New Classic Beauty

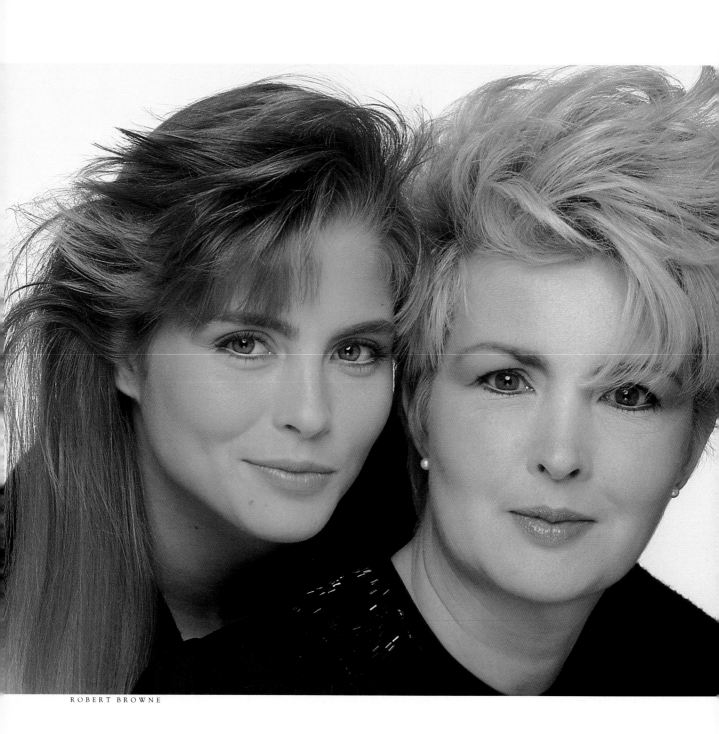

ROBERT BROWNE

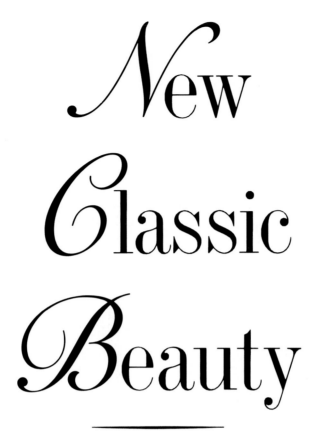

New Classic Beauty

A Step-by-Step Guide to

Naturally Glamorous

Makeup

by Joey Mills

Villard Books New York 1987

Library of Congress Catalogue Card Number:
87-040185

ISBN: 0-394-56433-2

Title page photo: Kim and Barbara Alexis—
Two Generations of Beauty

Designed by Iris Weinstein
Manufactured in the United States of America
9 8 7 6 5 4 3 2
First edition

To the loving memory of my mother, Doshie;
To my brother, Nathan, who is the source
  of my emotional strength;
To Mary and Carla Mills;
To Darnella Thomas.

Acknowledgments

I've been fortunate to work with the most talented photographers, models, hair stylists, magazine editors and creative directors. Many of them have generously contributed their time and talent to this book project.

I'm grateful to the following people for their help throughout my career: Kim Alexis, Sean Byrnes, Camille and Bill Cosby, the late Andre Douglas, Gloria Foster, Elaine Korn, Polly Mellen, Jay Mulford, Bert Padell, Andrea Robinson, Francesco Scavullo, Diane Smith, Susan Sommers, Martin Stevens, Rochelle Udell, Barry Weinbaum, Alvin Bell, and Hector Torres.

A special thanks to the following celebrities for allowing me the use of their images and the pleasure of working with them: Christie Brinkley, Phoebe Cates, Ruby Dee, Terry Farrell, Melissa Gilbert, Jessica Lange, Andie MacDowell, Liza Minnelli, Lee Remick, Isabella Rossellini, Brooke Shields, Shelley Smith, Barbara Walters.

Many thanks to the following photographers for the use of their photographs: Andrea Alberts, Paul Amato, George Barkentin, Howard Bingham, Eric Bowman, Robert Browne, Alex Chatelain, Michel Comte, Patrick Demarchelier, Les Goldberg, Horst, Ishimuro, Dominique Issermann, David King, Paul Lange, Klaus Laubmayer, Jimmy Moore, Ron Nicolaysen, Norman Parkinson, Denis Piel, Roger Prigent, Michael Raab, Michael Reinhardt, Francesco Scavullo, Frank E. Schramm III, John Stember, Shonna Valeska, Stan Wan, Albert Watson.

My thanks to all the beautiful models: Karen Alexander, Barbara Alexis, Kim Alexis, Carol Alt, Vanessa Angel, Susan Bearden, Bitten, Carmen, Nancy Donahue, Kelly Emberg, Dawn Gallagher, Debra Halley, Kristin "Clotilde" Holby, Iman, Beverly Johnson, Miky Kim, Carol Kurzin, Carey Lowell, Rosemary McGrowther, Deirdre McGuire, Kathy Martin, Terri-May, Amy Miles, Toni O'Reilly, Paulina Porizkova, Beth Rupert, Lisa Ryall, Rene Simonsen, Talisa Soto, Darnella Thomas, Maria von Hartz, Eva Voorhis, Julie Wolfe.

Thanks to the following hair stylists: John Atchison, Howard Fugler, Garren, Marc Pipino, Jonathan Roberson, John Sahag, Suga, Edward Tricome.

Thanks to all my friends at the model agencies for their help: Sue Charney of Sue Charney Models; Francis Grill and Allan Mindel of Click; Monique Pillard and Dottie Franco of Elite; Eileen, Jerry and Lacy Ford and Joey Hunter of the Ford Agency; Faith Kates and Karen Cohen of Wilhelmina; Susan Brannigan of Zoli.

Thanks to the following magazines and their editors for the use of their photographs: William Rayner, Diana Edkins and Conde Nast Publications; Linda Cox and *Cosmopolitan*; Michele Mazzola and *Harper's Bazaar*; Jim Franco and *Ladies' Home Journal*; Susan Reinhardt and *Redbook*.

Thanks to the following companies and their personnel: Freda Wein and Altman, Stoller, Weiss Advertising; Gail Blanke, Gary Kirschenbaum, Barry Weinbaum and Avon Products, Inc.; Jo Levin and Geer Gross Advertising; Joan Kennedy and Lancôme; Sheri Wilson-Gray and Monet; Allen Eichhorn and PMK Public Relations; Pat Goldberg and Ralph Lauren, Inc.; Alain Combe, Joel Schneider and Revlon, Inc.; Kimiko Kek-iguchi and Shu Uemura, Inc.; William Tuttle and William Tuttle, Inc.

With the help of my colleagues, I was able to combine the necessary elements to make this book instructive and fun to look at. But it is my good fortune to have as exceptional an editor as I have in Diane Reverand. Her guidance was instrumental in the final vision of this book.

Many thanks to Wendy Bass, Emily Bestler, Jessie Ristic and Iris Weinstein at Villard for their enthusiastic contributions.

I'd like to thank John Pirman for his line drawings.

Thanks to Candace Caldwell for all her help.

I'm twice blessed in my association with a very talented writer, Carolyn Fireside. Her writing captured all that I hoped for.

And finally, I'd like to thank Asher Jason, my literary agent and friend, for his continuing faith in me and my book. I'm deeply indebted to him for his advice and tenacity in making this book happen.

Contents

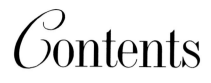

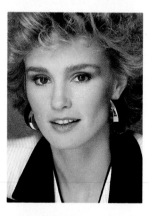
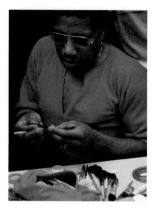
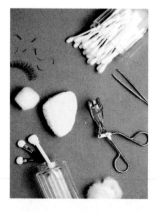
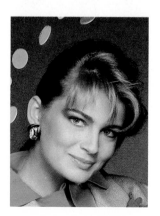
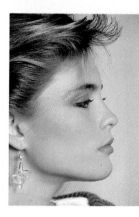

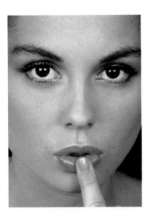
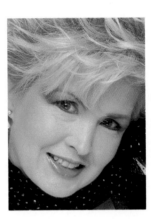
PART THREE • THE ONLY MAKEUP
GUIDE YOU'LL EVER NEED

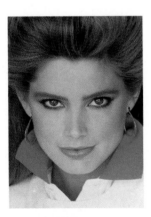
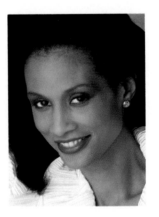
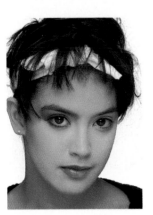

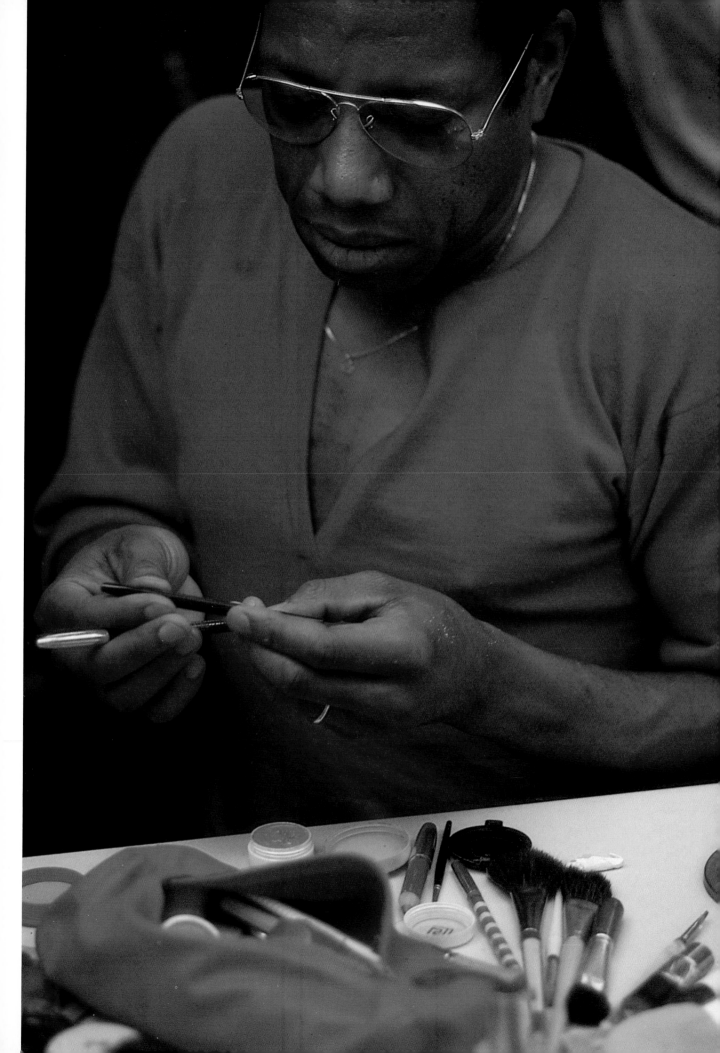

Introduction: Learning to Be Born Beautiful

New Classic Beauty—it's the look I love, the style I've devoted an entire career to perfecting. You've seen it on the cover of *Vogue*, on your favorite star in top makeup ads and fashion layouts, but I bet that most of the time you didn't notice that Barbara Walters or Jessica Lange was wearing makeup. You just noticed they looked beautiful—fresh, natural, glowing no matter what their age; wonderfully "finished" no matter what their facial flaws.

Here's the secret of their special appeal: They never looked more beautiful *and* they never looked more like themselves! They didn't look as if they were wearing masks on their faces. They radiated a healthy glow that comes from within, a serene self-confidence and an ease in being themselves. That's why you didn't notice the makeup. What you noticed was the enhancement of their natural glamour.

You, too, have natural glamour, a lot of it, and I don't want you camouflaging it behind red cheeks and aqua eyelids. No way! I'm going to show you how to be the best, the most elegant version of yourself you can be. I'm going to show you how to create the New Classic You!

Now, let's be frank about natural glamour and makeup. Although utterly unassisted beauty is what every woman dreams of, there really is no such thing. A woman wearing no makeup at all, even if she's a celebrated cover girl, is simply not making the most of her glamour potential. Doing the most with what you have is definitely the point for women these days. Look through the Before and After pictures in the pages that follow. You'll be astonished at the difference even light makeup can achieve.

I assure you that you won't, with my makeup system, go around looking like a copy of the latest cosmetic promotion or like everybody else, because the focus of New Classic Beauty is to enhance your individuality.

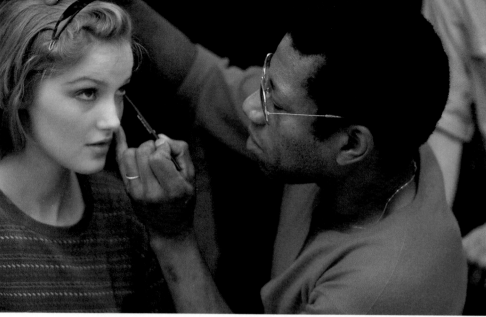

Whether you're on the slopes or in the wedding party, dancing all night or attending an all-day business meeting, you'll be able to devise and maintain your own personal look. As you study the instructions that follow and master my techniques, you'll be able to do a full makeup application in a mere sixteen minutes, even less to embellish or retouch. With practice, creating a radiant face will only take eight minutes of your valuable time! And you'll never, ever look exhausted or pressured, regardless of how tough your day—or night—has been.

Women who wear a lot of obvious makeup actually seem to wilt in the course of a couple of hours. Lipstick fades, eye shadow bleeds into creases, pencil liner or mascara smudges messily. You know. Even if these women aren't actually worn out, they look as if they are. With my classic "no makeup," the faded-flower syndrome is a thing of the past!

Now let's talk for a bit about individuality and the New Classic Beauty. Don't make the mistake of thinking that my system is only for sixteen-year-old, blue-eyed blondes—far from it. Lee Remick isn't sixteen and doesn't pretend to be. Isabella Rossellini and Debra Winger, who are neither blond nor blue-eyed, fit my classic style perfectly because of the easy and relaxed elegance of their looks. Diana Ross and Karen Alexander, who are black, certainly

personify natural glamour, as do redheads, exotic Hispanic and Asian women. Every woman has natural glamour. As a makeup artist, I capture your individualism, enhancing your natural aura and style.

The way to master beautiful makeup is not by following fashion or trying to reproduce a cosmetics ad that intrigues you. If the look is fabulous but not for you, it won't work. I believe that a woman can learn to know her face. But she must approach her makeup as she approaches her life—as her own very precious possession.

The key to New Classic Beauty is individuality and its expression, cleanness of line, subtlety of color and freshness. And, most of all, it's about having fun! I love to have fun, and I love my work. (When I was starting out, I had to choose between pro basketball and makeup. I drifted into makeup through modeling, and I found it gave me as great a high and presented as great a challenge as sports—and was a career that would last much longer—so I went for it.) I make certain my clients have a good time, too. While we're having fun creating the most beautiful "them" possible, we're also learning makeup tricks we'll continue to use long after the show or the shoot or the event is over.

Let's not kid ourselves: Learning to apply makeup correctly and flatteringly takes some effort and concentration at the beginning—no one ever said that getting control of your appearance was easy. Like everything else in life, it involves learning the rules, learning right from wrong.

"Wrong"—you've seen it too many times —is the shy girl who's trying to pass herself off as "hot," the middle-aged woman who's trying to look like her own daughter; the short, curvy woman with a round face who's trying to resemble Audrey Hepburn. "Wrong," literally, means too much of everything—mascara, rouge, liner and lipstick laid on with a trowel. "Right" means the correct shade of blush and well-blended foundation, a lighter hand with mascara and liner, a "stainy" mouth achieved without lip pencils. Remember, classic beauty is supposed to suggest, not shout to the world! And it'll only take you eight minutes, sixteen at first, but what's that compared to the pleasure you'll feel when people ask you if you've been on vacation or lost weight or if you're in love—they'll never guess that you've only changed your makeup.

I'm looking forward to sharing with you the secrets that have taken me fifteen years to develop, but, before we begin, here's the cornerstone of my technique: *color,* softly and subtly applied. I've even devised a series of color charts that will enable you to pick—without making expensive mistakes—the correct color tones for your individual hair, eye and skin colors. These charts are repeated at the end of the book on perforated paper so you can take your chart with you when you go makeup shopping and compare the colors to products before you buy them. The charts are the "magic wands" of my book. Not only will they tell you the colors you should choose, they'll also guide you to the right foundations, show you how to erase blemishes, skin discolorations and wrinkles as if they'd never been there, and guide you toward using your natural tonality as the jumping-off point for composing your face— eyes, cheeks, lips, hair, and skin, all done in marvelous harmony.

So read the instructions in the text and learn from the illustrations, all of which, I guarantee, are easy to follow. Study the personalized color charts. Then, sit yourself down at the little beauty area I want you to construct for yourself; well-lit, pleasingly decorated and arranged, it'll be a private nook where you can indulge in the healthy sensuality of bringing out your natural glamour.

I'm famous for styling the faces of the world's most beautiful women, and I can't wait to make you one of them!

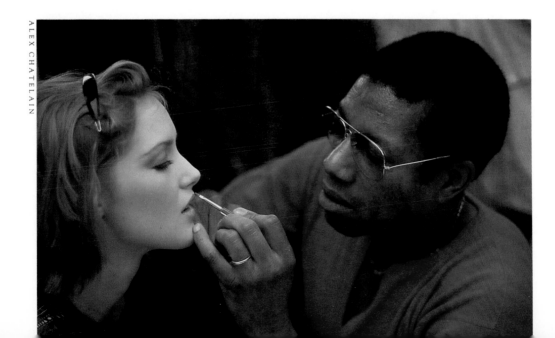

ALEX CHATELAIN

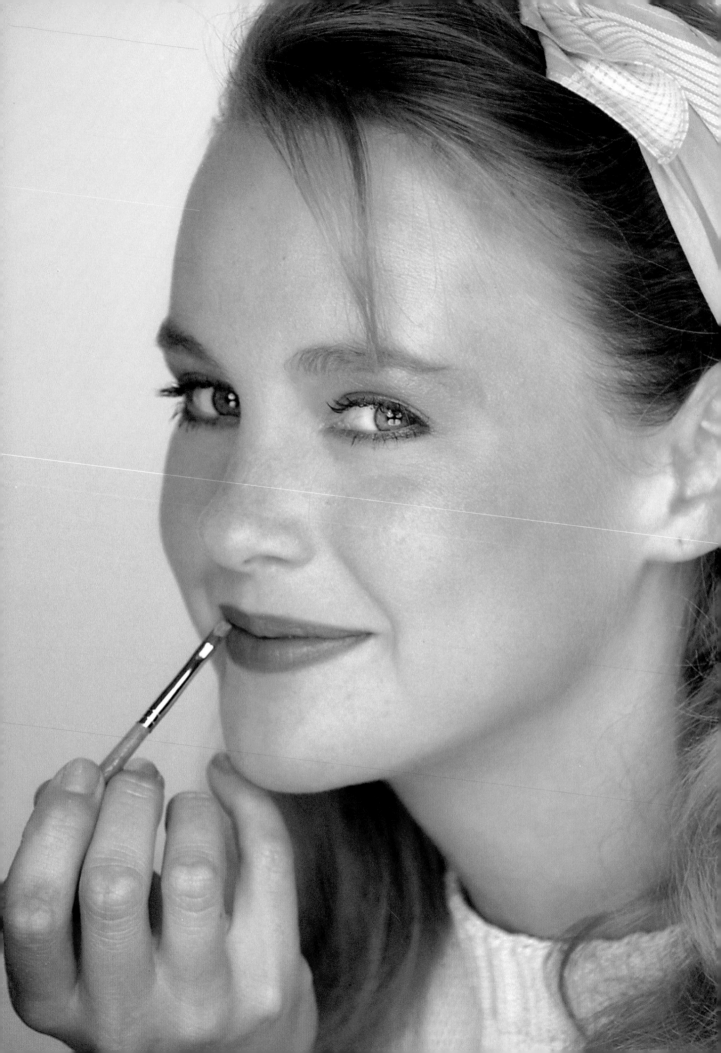

Part One

The Right Stuff

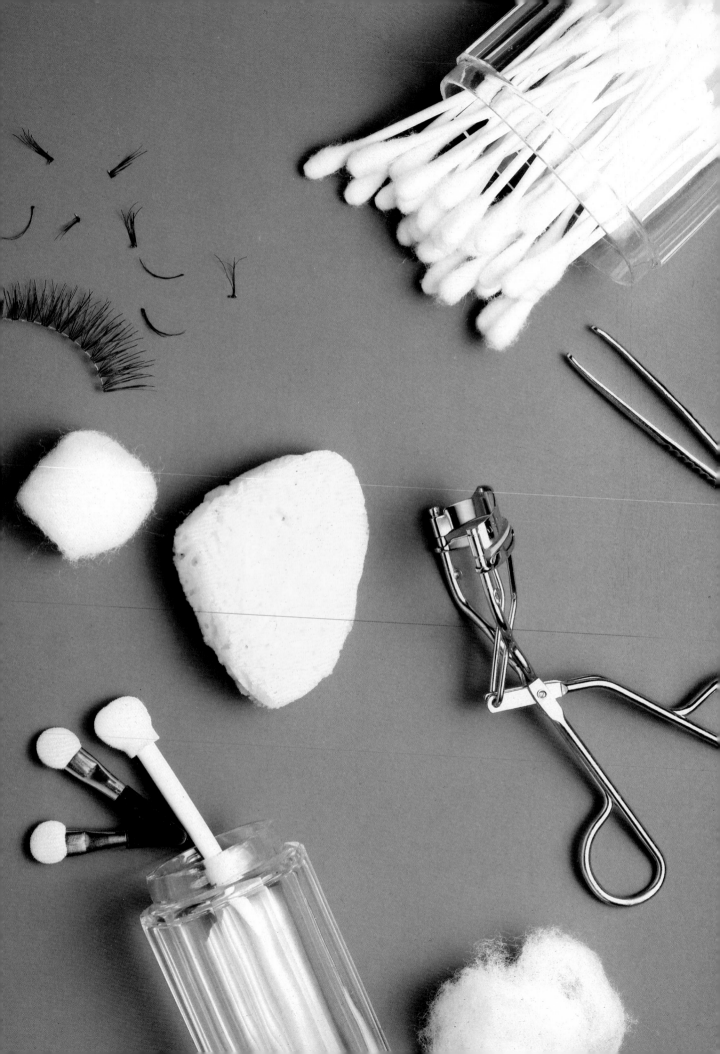

1

Every Woman's Tool Kit

Necessary Luxuries

The soft, sensual feel of a sable brush caressing your skin is one of life's great pleasures—after all, sable's sable, luxurious and always classic. Let me say right now, I believe in luxury, especially since my brand of luxury means sheer quality. Whether you're talking about a fur coat or a makeup brush, the luxury of an article that offers maximum performance over the long haul—a brush that keeps its shape or a coat that never goes out of style—is what "classic" is all about. "Classic" means ageless, a real luxury, and that's what I'm offering: the New Classic You regardless of years or tiny, correctable flaws. You deserve quality, you deserve luxury—remember that. And a little self-indulgence, especially when it doesn't have to be replaced as often and so ends up being economical, never hurt anybody. Now, let's get on to an area of makeup where luxury is essential: the tools you'll be working with, from brushes through tweezers to my personalized, portable color charts!

The importance of
essentials

Brushes and Other Musts

*B*rushes are modulators. You'll shade with them, blend with them, understate with them until you execute the strokes without thinking about it—lightly and with great skill. They're the agents of cosmetic subtlety, the very essence of the New Classic Look as opposed to staginess.

Whatever you do, don't scrimp on brushes. It simply is not worth it. All you get in a "bargain" brush is hairs that will shed on your face, an applicator that doesn't hold its shape—in short, more trouble than the item's worth.

Listen, if you've ever been intimidated by one of those exquisitely packaged sets of cosmetic brushes (What could they all be *for?*), you're not alone. Most people aren't professional makeup artists, actresses or models, and so they haven't had occasion to learn. But I'm going to do something about that right now.

A well-equipped makeup table doesn't have to look like Van Gogh's studio, which is to say you don't have to assemble a huge collection of brushes. In fact, you need only five or six, but they have to be of good quality so they won't shed or lose their shape. They must travel well—be able to fit in a purse or a weekender—and they have to be washable.

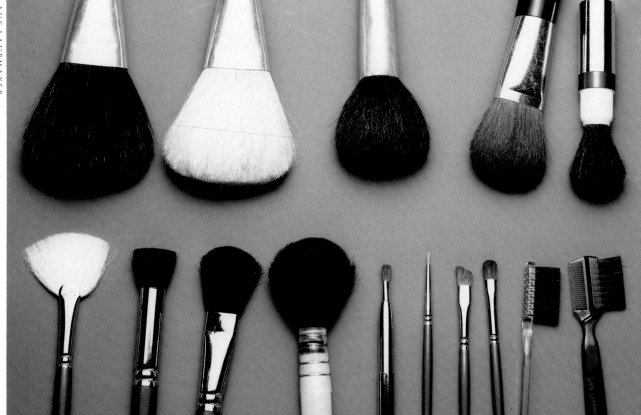

THE ESSENTIAL
COMPLEXION BRUSHES ARE:

Powder brush
Shading brush
Color brush
Cleanup brush
Slimming brush
Cover-up brush
Natural silk sponge
(not a brush, but
serves a version of the
same function)

The Powder Brush

You'll be using this for "dusting off" the loose powder you'll have applied over foundation or moisturizer to prepare the "canvas" of your face for eye, cheek and lip makeup.

Why Use a Powder Brush?

For silky, transluscent skin, after dabbing on powder with a puff (over base or moisturizer), use the brush to dust off the excess. What you'll get is a guarantee that your makeup won't look cakey, yet it will still provide enough coverage to prevent the oil in your skin from emerging and creating the dreaded "shine." So, to avoid the "shine" as long as possible, use the powder brush to dust off the loose powder that you've applied with the puff.

The Shading and Color Brushes

These tools are used in tandem to give your face a subtle glow.

Brushes: tricks of the trade
TOP, LEFT TO RIGHT:
A domed dark sable brush to dust off powder from your face. A body brush to add highlight powder to neck, shoulders, bare skin. A color brush to blend color. A rouge brush to apply powder rouge; it's slightly stiffer than the oversized brushes, which I prefer, but some women prefer a smaller brush. That clean-up brush to use under your eyes when eye shadow falls or flakes; it cleans up undereye area without smudging or rubbing.

BOTTOM, LEFT TO RIGHT:
Another clean-up brush —my second choice, but I included it and it's generally available wherever brushes are sold, from the five-and-ten to Bloomingdale's. A classic contour brush with a flat, blunt edge for cheeks, temples, forehead, and sides of neck (if you're wearing a low-cut gown). A brush to apply a little bit of color. If you have very pale skin and you've done your rouge but you still look white around the eyes, use this brush—deep red into a little of pale peach-colored rouge to add color

or to soften around the eyes. Another clean-up powder brush that can also be used with shimmer powder; it's your little "powder puff." A very thin retractable lip brush to use when applying lipstick for moisture only.

Always use a brush. It makes lipstick last longer.

A classic eyelining brush to apply "optional" eye colors (see chart).

Never use the applicator that comes with eye shadows to apply eye shadow; it's for blending

out eye shadow only. Skip eyeliner pencils too— they're not soft or subtle enough. A nose shading brush with a wedged edge for the ends of your nose. A softening brush to take away any hard lines, blend out your eye shadow to soften any lines. An eyebrow brush to use on naturally unarched brows. A classic combination comb/brush with one side for eyelashes, to comb or brush through excess mascara, a brush for brows.

Why Use Color and Shading Brushes?

You'll be applying a bronzer rouge, also called shading powder, with the shading brush, to enhance the shape of your face and accentuate your cheekbones. Over that you'll add cheek color (brighter rouge) using the color brush, which will add vibrancy to your skin tone. The color brush is used to blend the shading powder with the brighter rouge to produce the classic "no makeup" cheek.

The Cleanup Brush

This priceless treasure can save you endless time by correcting mistakes without your having to start over.

Why Use a Cleanup Brush?

Any smudges of eye liner or shadow that happen to land where they shouldn't can be banished with a light flick of the cleanup brush. And it won't leave little red marks on your face or smudge your makeup.

The Slimming Brush

Less basic and more sophisticated than the other brushes, the uses of this valuable tool will be more thoroughly explained when I discuss face contouring. This flat, thin brush, when used around the jawline, literally slims. Used correctly, it takes "ten pounds" off an overly full face.

The Cover-up Brush

When you master the art of this little gem, you'll think you've discovered a miracle.

Why Use a Cover-up Brush?

With this you'll be applying cover-up under eyes and over laugh lines to correct any lines, hidden valleys or facial imperfections. And after a rough day or a long night, this implement, when used with camouflage creme or powder under and around the eyes, minimizes puffiness and makes you look alert and well rested.

Natural Silk Sponge

Last, but not least, is the brush that isn't a brush. Although rubbery sponges are much easier to find, I always opt for the natural silk. Rubbery sponges can cause skin to break out and I'm a cleanliness addict: Just as you should wash your brushes (which is one important reason to use sable with level bristles), you should and must wash your sponge—almost every time you use it.

Why Use a Natural Silk Sponge?

There's nothing better with which to apply and even out foundation. Never use your fingers because you'll be adding oil to your face (and encouraging "shine"); you'll also be tugging at your skin with your fingers and getting foundation under your fingernails.

Eye Contact

*B*efore you even begin to try to achieve New Classic Beauty, you're going to have to have some supplies.

THE ESSENTIAL EYE TOOLS ARE:
A very, very thin eyeliner brush
Sponge applicators
Cotton swabs
Eyelash curler
Eyelash comb and brush
Eyebrow brush/comb for lashes
A tweezer

Eyeliner Brush

I call this the "cheating brush" because it's the thinnest and finest of all basic brushes, and it can do the most with the least.

Why Use an Eyeliner Brush?

I'll tell you in detail in Chapter 4, but suffice it to say that lining your eyes, both top and bottom, then learning how to smudge is the essence of New Classic Beauty. You'll learn how to use the brush to do this procedure using either wet or dry eye shadows.

Sponge Applicators

The applicators that come with eye shadow love to be skimpy so they can fit in the com-pacts. I prefer a larger applicator, so I recommend you pick up a package of little sponges on sticks. They're reasonably priced, come in packs of four or so and are easier to use —effectively.

Cotton Swabs

Among the mortal sins committed against makeup is the hard line around the eyes. I'm mad about shadowing, but not so the woman looks like an ancient Egyptian statue; around the eye, liner should be subtly applied and artfully smudged.

Why Use a Cotton Swab?

I'll show you how to master the art of smudging in Chapter 4, but be aware that cotton swabs are also invaluable in correcting and cleaning up mistakes. However, be careful that you maintain a very light touch so as to avoid irritating or reddening the skin.

The Eyelash Curler

You'll be surprised at how quickly this tool becomes indispensable; not only will it make lashes look longer and more natural, it will make them healthier and stronger.

Why Use an Eyelash Curler?

Gently grip upper lashes, as close to the base as possible, then roll the curler upward before releasing the lashes. Make sure you do this before you apply mascara.

The Eyelash Comb/ Eyebrow Brush

Essential for creating natural looking brows and lashes, these tools often come as "a combo," in one implement.

Why Use an Eyelash Comb?

After applying your mascara, draw the teeth of the comb through your lashes to prevent them from clumping. Next, apply a second coat of mascara, then comb the lashes again: I guar-antee your eyelashes will never have looked as luscious and natural.

Why Use an Eyebrow Brush?

Expertise with this simple but invaluable tool will give you the lush, orderly brows you've always dreamed of. After you've applied your eye makeup, shape your brows by brushing the hairs of your brow upward and over to form a natural arch.

Tweezers

I recommend using the slanted style because it captures stray hairs more efficiently. And, remember, you're using the tweezers to prune, not to create an artificial shape. What you don't want is a brow tweezed to one narrow, harsh line.

Lip Service

THE ESSENTIAL LIP TOOLS ARE:

Lipstick brush   Sharpener

Lipstick Brush

This tool is an absolute necessity and should be carried with you at all times! Applying lipstick directly from the tube is a major no-no because it's just plain wasteful. Good for the cosmetic companies, bad for your budget! By the way, that applies to glosses, too. Not only does a brush actually conserve the amount of lipstick or gloss you use at a time, but it also

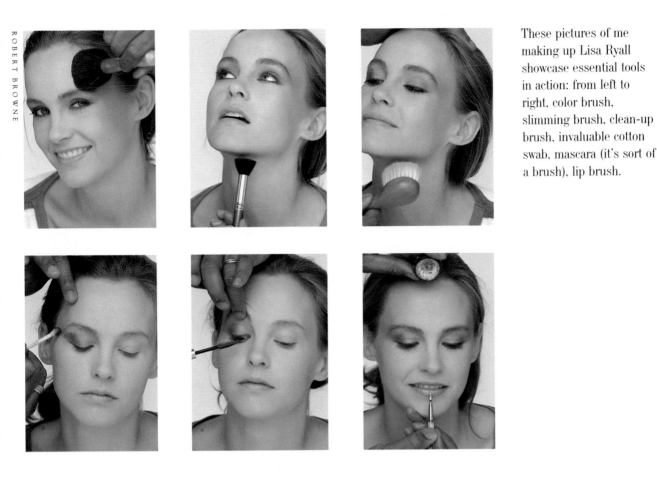

ROBERT BROWNE

These pictures of me making up Lisa Ryall showcase essential tools in action: from left to right, color brush, slimming brush, clean-up brush, invaluable cotton swab, mascara (it's sort of a brush), lip brush.

allows you to use one color to achieve different looks—from transparent to opaque, from sheer to matte, even the lovely subtle look of a slight stain.

Why Use a Lipstick Brush?

Stroke the brush across your lips, just a couple of times for minimal coverage. If you want more vibrant, intense lips, simply stroke on more, but very gradually. If you "take up" too much color for your lips, just blot off the excess with a tissue. (My secret lip tip: If you really want to achieve the "satiny" look, don't use lipstick at all; use two lip pencils, blended. I'll show you exactly how to get this effect in Chapter 6.)

Pencil Sharpener

Tiny but powerful, the sharpener is definitely a must. Here's a tip: Since many cosmetic pencils have soft "lead," place them in the freezer and let them harden before you sharpen them.

Last Words About Brushes

*D*on't conserve on quality where brushes are concerned because you'll end up being penny-wise and pound-foolish. Good brushes actually last longer, and they won't shed. Your safest bet are animal-hair bristles, and the top of that line are the models that use inner hairs, which are softer. Brushes labeled "sensitive skin" are made from the downiest hairs so that the bristles will slide across the skin without the risk of irritation or tugging.

What you're looking for in a makeup brush is that it be nonirritating and nontugging, that it not shed, that it retain its shape and not splay out. The more tightly packed the hairs the better, because it means the brush will do a good job of grabbing and holding onto color. Before you buy any brush, play with it to be sure it will retain its shape.

How to Care for Your Brushes

Every few weeks, brushes must be washed with mild, liquid soap and water. Just fill a basin with water, add soap and swish the brushes around until all color is removed. Mold the wet brush back into its original shape, then rest it on a towel to dry overnight. It'll come out as good as new—and last for years!

Getting Good at It

By the time you finish studying this book and have practiced the sixteen-minute makeup and its even shorter variations, you'll be surprised by the flexibility you've developed with brushes, with tweezers, with the whole battery of tools. Soon, the flexibility will become second nature.

So, now that you've gotten a good grounding in using the applicators, you're ready to go on to what you'll apply with them: color.

RON NICOLAYSEN

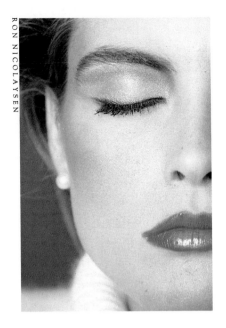 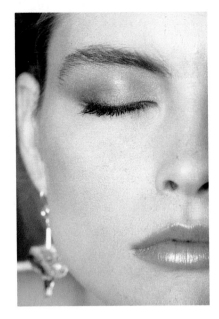

Kim Alexis:
Right and Wrong
When I tell you light is
right, you'll believe me
after comparing these
pictures of Kim Alexis.

The photo on the left
has the eye done utterly
wrong. Look at it. Not
only are the three eye
shadows not blended in
the least, but they clash.
In addition to everything
else, the shadow was
applied so haphazardly
that it's unrelated to the
beautiful shape of the eye.
Gad!

The photo on the left is, if
I say so myself, a vast
improvement. See how
the subtle blending of
colors enhances the
eyelid, and the way it
sweeps outward and up,
lifting her entire face.

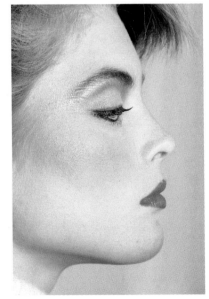 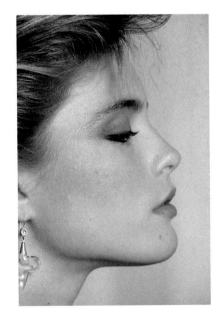

The photo on the left is
totally taboo. How could
anybody do this to a
beautiful woman like
Kim? All you see is
cheeks and lips bursting
away from the face. All
you see is the
exaggerated features and
color. In addition to
downplaying her natural
beauty, this makeup,
frankly, makes even Kim
look tacky.

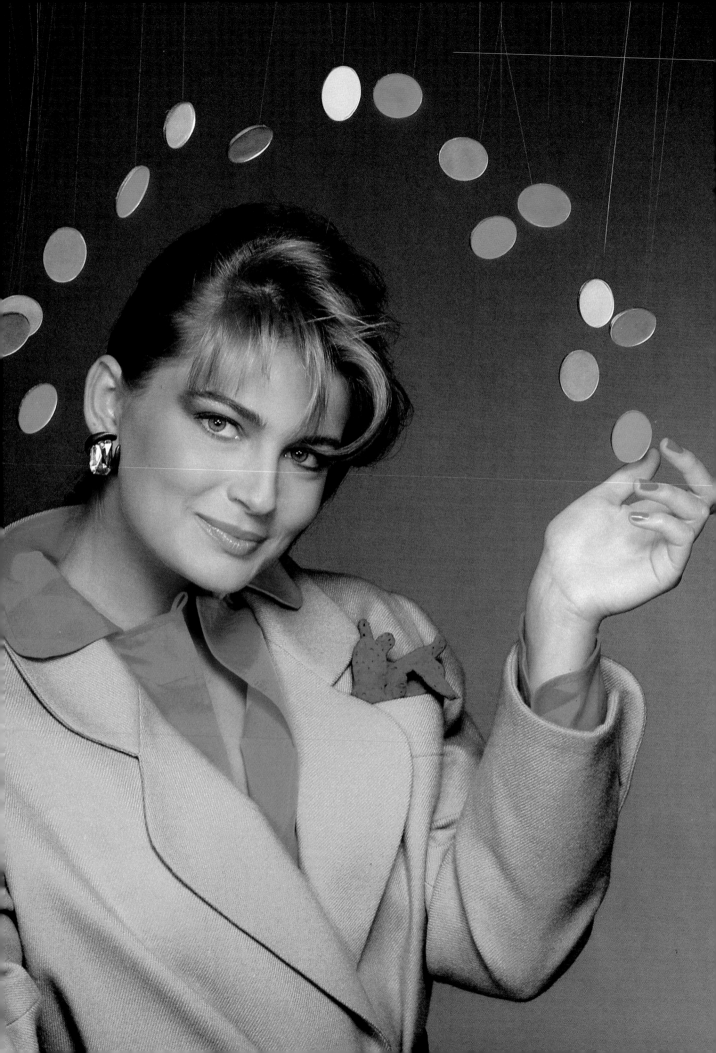

2

Your Personal Color Scheme
(and My Individual Color Charts)

Let's Call a Halt to Makeup Madness

To err with an occasional lipstick is human; to choose perfect colors every time is divine, and, believe me, you'll be doing it soon! All you need is the right information, including a good knowledge and appreciation of your personal color scheme.

Of course you've made silly cosmetics mistakes in the past. Everyone, at one time or another, has fallen for an irresistible cosmetics campaign, run to the nearest counter and charged up quite a bill for a "complete" look. But once you were away from the hypnotic power of department store lighting and shopping frenzy, it became obvious that all the stuff actually *clashed* with the colors of your hair,

eyes and skin. Those days are over forever.

I'm going to teach you how to select colors that always coordinate—with your skin, your eyes, your hair, even your eyeglass frames, and, for evening, with your outfit. The "finished" look that is essential to the New Classic Beauty really means perfect coordination. And I'm not talking about "matching." That's a bad fashion mistake. Wearing the same pink on your lips as is in your sweater is a major no-no! So is a dark green evening gown and dark green liner! Remember, always "coordinate." It's essential; you must do it even when it means passing up a gorgeous product because it doesn't go with your color scheme.

Paulina Porizkova
Color: the key to New
Classic Beauty

My Ultrasecret Color Charts— Revealed for the First Time!

*E*veryone (including makeup artists) haunts the makeup counters looking for the new, the truly different, the unexpected, but to be honest, we usually don't find it. And with good reason: In the world of cosmetics and makeup, especially classic makeup, there really isn't, nor should there be, anything radically new under the sun. (Black lipstick and red mascara are novelty items and don't count.)

A color is a color. No matter what a manufacturer calls a certain color—this one's "putty" may be that one's "mushroom"—you can find any color in most cosmetic lines under another name and with only the slightest variation. Even when shades vary, what always stays the same is the tone, the essence of a particular color.

To guide you through the jungle of exotic names and miraculous claims, I'm giving you color charts for your specific hair, eye and skin tones. There are seven charts in all. Two apply to everyone: foundations and evening colors. The others are for specific types: brunettes, blondes, redheads, gray-haired women and exotics. In the pages ahead, you can glance at the charts that apply to you and see the colors that will work for you. Then, when you're ready to go out and buy what you need, turn to the back of the book where an identical series of charts can be torn out. Take these with you to the store and actually match the color you'll be buying to the color I've recommended. Before each chart, I'll talk you through your individual colors and even suggest a few extras that don't appear on the charts.

Remember, knowing the *name* of the color is less important than being able to recognize the appropriate *tone*.

A Few Words About Using the Colors You Choose

Eye Color—the Triple Threat

I always use shadow in three different but equally important ways: (1) as shadow, in its dry, natural form; (2) as eyeliner, wet and applied with a fine eyeliner brush; (3) as an eye contourer. I favor dark shades of shadow. Not only does this technique ensure a fresh, natural look, but it's also economical because you won't go through the shadow as fast. As with all of New Classic Beauty, I'm not suggesting you go out and buy everything in the makeup department. What I'm suggesting is that you buy the *right* essentials, and not a lot of them, only those that will be multipurpose and never go out of style. Here's a great tip: If you can't find the exact color you want, you can achieve it by blending either gray or brown, gray to blue and green tones, brown to red and earth tones.

Cheeky Glamour

To find the right colors of blusher, check the hair charts, which give you two classic colors; basic and foolproof, they'll always work. The other five colors offered are chosen on the basis of your eye color and can be used alone as color or to add punch right on top of one of the classics. Which "addition" you opt for really is up to you, as long as it's coordinated with your eye color and blended out over the classic so no one can see that they were ever two different colors.

Lip Smarts

I prefer lip pencils over lipstick a thousand to one because I like the look of a matte finish that doesn't come off on a wine glass or on a cheek when you kiss someone.

Where color selection is concerned, my lip color charts are geared to your hair and eye tones. Cinnamon, however, appears on every chart because it's right for every woman—as a base tone. (The exception to this iron-clad rule is dark-skinned women who might want to think about a darker, almost black pencil or contour cream to even out lips that may actually be two-toned—a light bottom lip and a lighter top one.)

Enchanted Evenings

I want to tell you about a new generation of product that will transform you into a fairy-tale princess in seconds. It's called shimmer powder, and it's truly the makeup equivalent of fairy dust. When you're dressed for a night of splendor—your gown is perfect, your hair is elegance itself, your makeup is classic but beautifully defined—go for the magic! Shimmer powder!

This marvelous evening invention comes last in the makeup process. Available in a range of lovely hues (as you'll see in the color charts) from silver, gold and bronze through fuchsia and slate, shimmer powders are coordinated with what you're wearing. They're meant to cast a warm, alluring aura. The last thing you'll do before you depart for the ball is take up your powder brush and dust lightly over your cheeks, eyes, even lips. But don't stop there. If your dress is strapless or sleeveless or low cut, lightly dust the powder over your shoulders and collar bones.

Coordination is such a personal thing and so central to your individual style that I'm going to give you permission to choose your own shimmer powder, based on what you're wearing. You don't want to match—that's a major fashion taboo—but you do want to coordinate. For instance, if you're wearing a strapless rose-red dress, you wouldn't want to use a red shimmer powder, even if they made one; you'd want a tone that "clicks" with your outfit. If you want to bring out the blue in the rose, use slate. If you want to highlight the orangy-gold in a bright red dress, you might opt for gold. See what I mean? You'll be striving for shimmer, not shine; for impression, not announcement.

Designing yourself for evening is creating yourself as a work of art. And shimmer powder is definitely the finishing touch.

Now let's get to the good stuff—the charts themselves.

Charting Your Color Course

*O*nce you see how useful these are, and how easy they are to master, you'll never want to be parted from them. Here's how they work. Let's say you're a hazel-eyed, medium brunette with light but not alabaster skin and, on this particular day, a pimple on your cheek.

• You'll choose the color of your undertoner according to your skin tone type and always apply it with a cover-up brush. In this case, choose classic turquoise cover toner. It will work for all skin tones (including exotic) except extra fair, which takes green tone. Foundation, which is always matched to the skin on your neck (this is the one time it's essential to match), is listed according to natural skin tones. Looking at the sample under brunette in the color chart, you surmise you're not very fair, but your skin isn't olive. That probably means you're in the second group of foundations—light beige and light medium beige. Let's talk frankly: You're going to have to invest in two foundations, but you'll know, with the color chart, exactly which two they should be no matter what the brand name is. When you get them home, retire to your makeup area and, on a piece of white paper, keep trying to blend different combinations of the two until you get one that matches the skin on your neck.

The match, we're assuming, is based on either winter or summer. Clearly, your skin changes when you spend more time out of doors, so in the winter you'll probably require more light beige, and in the summer you'll add more light medium beige.

• Undereye cream is pretty basic, available in two tints, one for light to medium, the other for medium to dark skin. You'll take the lighter of the two because you fall in the less exotic half of the chart.

Turning to the page that reads "Brunettes, Eyes," you'll see three basic colors which work for all brunettes regardless of eye color. Of the three basic tones, you'll be using rust and bronze as shadow and slate as liner.

• In addition, I'm giving you the optional colors, which are keyed to the color of your eyes. In this case, your optional selections are mushroom, a soft gray to bring out the green in your irises and perhaps a navy liner to highlight the gold flecks and brown tones.

• Moving on to cheek color, here again you'll find two classic colors for all brunettes and five others geared to eye color. Among the classics, you've picked a soft red, then, from the optionals, copper for contouring under color.

• Lip-wise, you look under "Lips Brunette" and find a mixture of classics and eye-coordinated optionals, plus a gold shimmer powder that you'll mix with lip gloss and use on your lower lip in the evening. You'll take the two basic lip pencils for day, the utterly classic cinnamon and sienna tones, but you're also tempted by a translucent mauve that is geared to hazel eyes.

A tip about evening: Remember, shimmer color is always coordinated with what you're wearing. Let's say your dress is ice blue. Since at night the outfit is the starring feature, your makeup makes a similar but slightly stronger statement than it does during the day. So you'll use slate-gray blue to line your eyes; instead of eye shadow, you'll use a warm but subtle color blush, and you'll be keeping your mouth pale. Now just before you're ready to leave, brush on a pearlized shimmer, which will bring out the sparkle of the ice in the blue.

That's the master example for a hazel-eyed, medium-pale brunette. Here are the variations that apply to you personally.

Foundation from A to Z

Undertones

Green Tone—
the fairest of skins

Turquoise—
the class undertoner
for all skin tones

Highlights
undereye cover

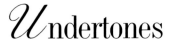

Light medium

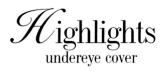

Medium to dark

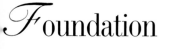 oundation

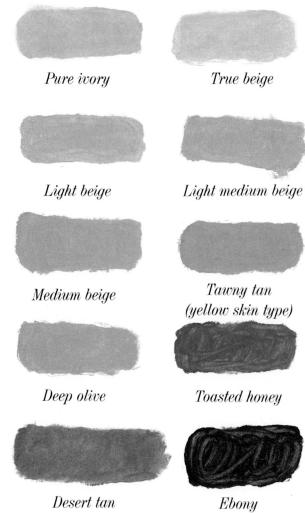

Pure ivory   *True beige*

Light beige   *Light medium beige*

Medium beige   *Tawny tan*
                                 (yellow skin type)

Deep olive   *Toasted honey*

Desert tan   *Ebony*   *Chocolate*

If You're a Brunette

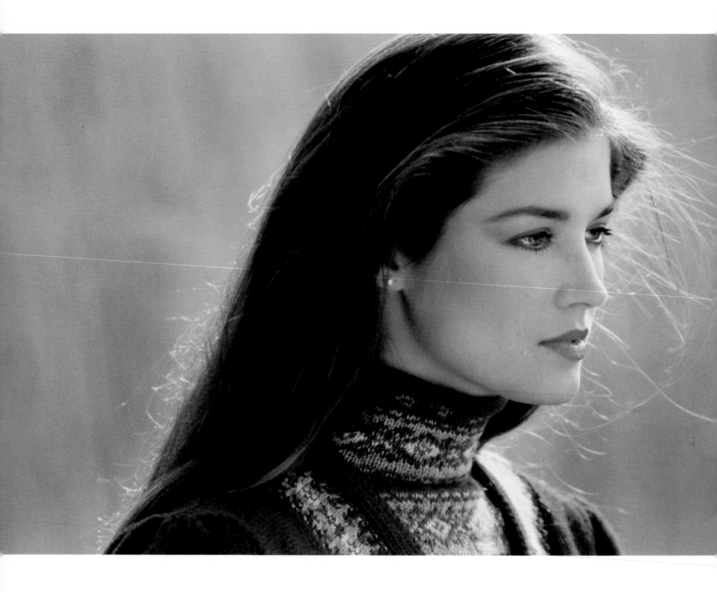

This is Clotilde, who typifies New Classic Beauty for brunettes. It's a famous photo, a ground-breaking picture, and it comes pretty close to defining New Classic Beauty. So many tones; so few bright, clashing colors. All you really see is Clotilde, lovely to look at. Her look is so fall she makes you feel that it's always the first semester and it's going to be a great year!

Foundation Color for Brunettes

If you're very pale, blend pure ivory and light beige; if medium light, light beige to light medium beige; if you're olive, medium beige to tawny; if you're darker or have a tan, deep olive to toasted honey.

Eye Color for Brunettes

Your three basic shadows are rust, bronze and slate. Your optionals, for shadowing and lining, depend on eye color; classic brown for blue eyes, soft gray for green eyes, mushroom for hazel eyes, navy for brown eyes and olive for dark brown eyes.

Cheek Color for Brunettes

You can take more intensity than your blonde sisters, but don't get carried away. Although the tones of your makeup may be stronger, they must be applied just as softly. Your classic cheek colors are sandalwood and peach (check the chart for the most flattering cheek color to go with your eyes). Everyone will do their contouring with copper.

Lip Color for Brunettes

Here, again, more color, but not a lot. Classic sienna and caramel and a clear red for evening look great on the whole world, as does tawny pink. You ought to have them in your collection. The chart includes lip colors to complement your eyes. For evening, mix shimmer powder in the gold range with your lip gloss and apply it to your bottom lip to give it the illusion of a sexy pout that makeup pros call a "roll."

Brunettes

Eyes

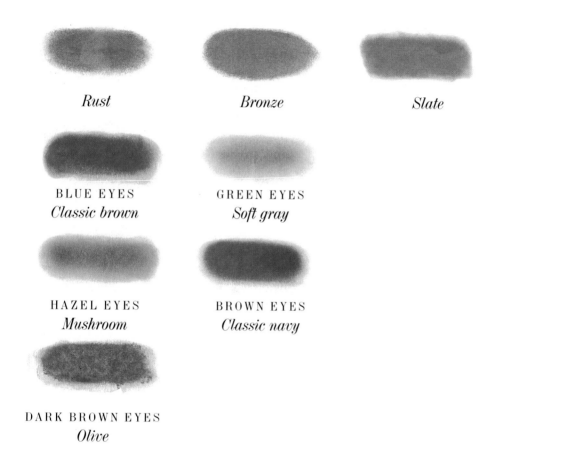

Rust　　　　　*Bronze*　　　　　*Slate*

BLUE EYES
Classic brown

GREEN EYES
Soft gray

HAZEL EYES
Mushroom

BROWN EYES
Classic navy

DARK BROWN EYES
Olive

*C*heeks   *L*ips

Sandalwood

Peach

Cinnamon

Sienna

BLUE EYES
Cinnamon

GREEN EYES
Tawny

BLUE EYES
Coral

GREEN EYES
Clear red

HAZEL EYES
Toasty tan blush

BROWN EYES
Grape tan

HAZEL EYES
Tawny pink

BROWN EYES
Rose/Pink

DARK BROWN EYES
Mauve rouge

DARK BROWN EYES
Garnet

If You're a Blonde

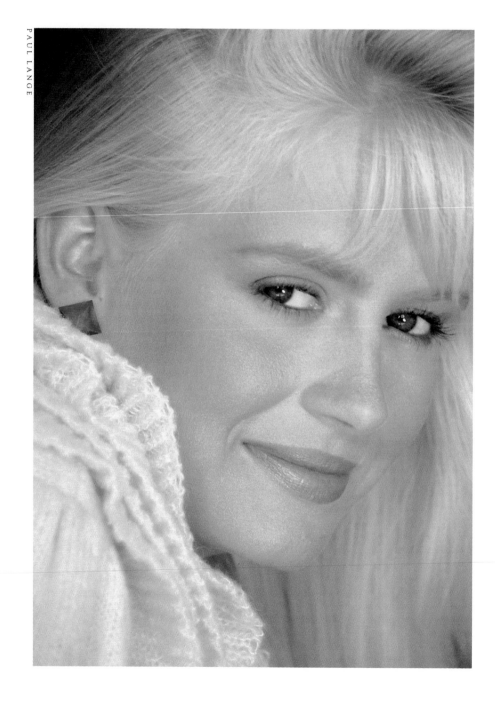

PAUL LANGE

Bitten is definitely the blonde on blonde in my portfolio. She's like peaches and cream, early summer, not tan, still palest gold. Isn't she lovely? The tribute to both of us is that she has the bone structure and I have a way with color. Examine the picture closely. See how much is makeup.

Foundation Color for Blondes

If your skin is very light, you'll be blending pure ivory and true beige. The blend depends on whether or not you have a tan. If your skin is medium light, blend light and light medium beige.

Eye Color for Blondes

All three of your basic tones are in the gold family—light gold or dark gold or sunny terracotta—while the five optionals offer variety as shadow or liner. Golds work for any shade of blonde, so you're going to have to take your eye color into account before making a final selection.

Blondes, no matter what shade their hair, have to keep in mind that the hair is always the star and makeup the accessory, more so than for any other hair color. What I'm saying is don't overdo your makeup to take attention away from your hair; it won't work. If you want to "frame" your eyes and give them more punch, line them with any of the shadows in the chart, always applied wet. And please, stay away from black! It's just plain gauche.

Cheek Color for Blondes

Here, too, your hair is the star. You don't want your face to be colorless, but you've got to keep it very understated. For your cheeks, soft bronze or a classic peach are right. Check your color chart to find the most flattering cheek color to go with your eyes.

For contouring, and to use your color blush, you should use a dark bronze, applied very subtly, regardless of eye color.

Lip Color for Blondes

Once more, keep it light, using the classic cinnamon or sienna. For brown eyes, a pastel coral, soft garnet or wood rose is flattering; for dark brown eyes, try golden cider; for blue or green eyes, take a chance with beigy pink.

For platinum blondes with blue, green or hazel eyes, I recommend a pale peach.

And for everyone, I recommend mixing gold shimmer powder with lip gloss as a finisher for your bottom lip in the evening.

Blondes

Eyes

Light gold

Dark gold

Terra-cotta

BLUE EYES
Slate

GREEN EYES
Classic peacock

HAZEL EYES
Mustard brown

BROWN EYES
Classic burgundy

DARK BROWN EYES
French blue

Cheeks

Soft bronze

Classic peach

BLUE EYES
Cinnamon

GREEN EYES
Creamy cocoa

HAZEL EYES
Sandalwood

BROWN EYES
Pale mauve

DARK BROWN EYES
Sienna

Lips

Cinnamon

Sienna

BLUE EYES
Natural beige pink

GREEN EYES
Classic clear pink

HAZEL EYES
Pale peach

BROWN EYES
Wood rose

DARK BROWN EYES
Golden cider

If You're a Redhead

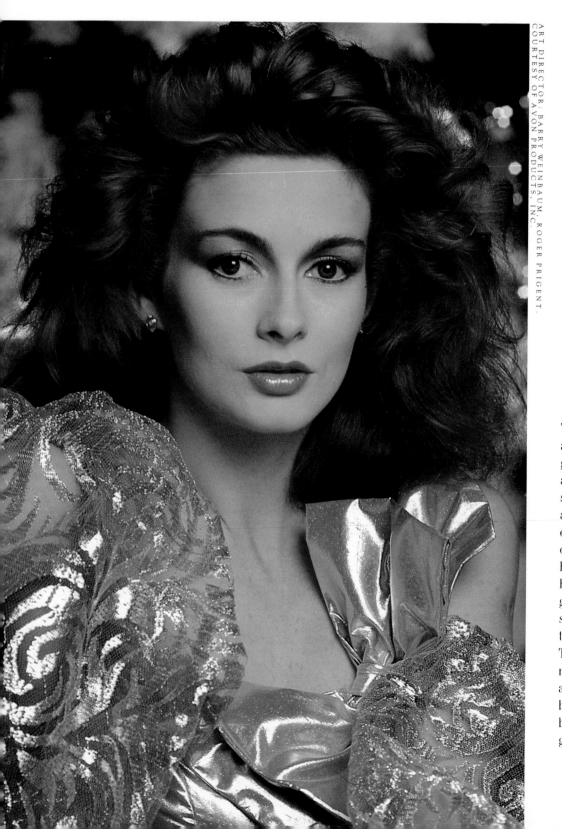

ART DIRECTOR: BARRY WEINBAUM, ROGER PRIGENT. COURTESY OF AVON PRODUCTS, INC.

Toni O'Reilly is the absolute epitome of a gorgeous redhead—look at the perfect match of skin and hair, apricots and cool fire. In this evening shot, notice that I coordinated the gold of her dress with the gold of her eye shadow to give a golden burnish that serves as a great contrast to the blaze of her hair. The mouth has color, but not overpowering, and it's also in a contrasting burnish. The peachy blush contributes a softer, gentler flame.

Foundation Color for Redheads

If you're very light, blend pure ivory and true beige; medium light, blend light beige and light medium beige, depending on whether or not you have a tan.

Eye Color for Redheads

Because your hair is so shocking and such an attention-getter, you must make sure to build your makeup around subtle and powdery blended color, not hard or definite. Please, no jade greens or vibrant blues, which will fight with your hair in the worst possible way.

All the colors on your chart are in the olive/taupe range, and the three basic shadows apply to every redhead regardless of eye color: viridian, cinnamon and soft charcoal—always softly blended. Optional colors for specific eye colors appear on the chart, and all can be used either dry as shadow or wet as liner.

Cheek Color for Redheads

A word of warning: Redheads with freckles *cannot* use a blush that contains any red because the red will enhance what you want to downplay. Classic redhead cheek colors are either beige matte blush or cinnamon. Your chart shows optional colors to coordinate with your eyes. For every redhead, dark bronze is preferred for contouring.

Lip Color for Redheads

Remember, lip color is coordinated with eyes, not hair, and the classic lip colors for redheads are sienna and cinnamon. Lip colors to complement your eyes are found on the chart. For evening, you'll want to use shimmer powder mixed with lip gloss on the bottom lip for a little sexy poutiness.

Redheads

Eyes

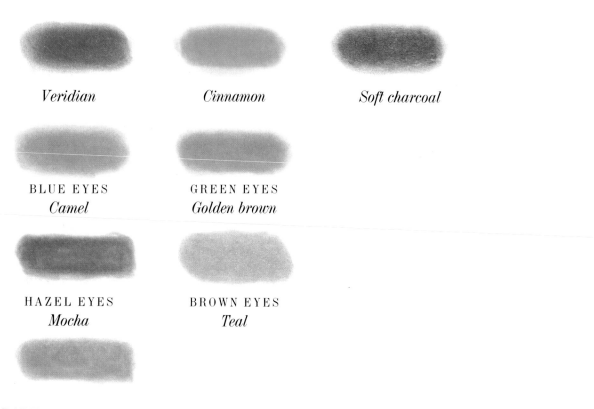

Veridian　　　　*Cinnamon*　　　　*Soft charcoal*

BLUE EYES
Camel

GREEN EYES
Golden brown

HAZEL EYES
Mocha

BROWN EYES
Teal

DARK BROWN EYES
Teal

*C*heeks

*L*ips

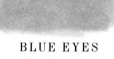

Beige matte blush

Cinnamon

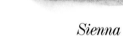

Sienna

Cinnamon

BLUE EYES
Sandalwood

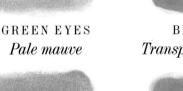

GREEN EYES
Pale mauve

BLUE EYES
Transparent bordeaux

GREEN EYES
Clear soft peach

HAZEL EYES
Tawny rouge

BROWN EYES
Silky mauve

HAZEL EYES
Gold copper

BROWN EYES
Peach bronze

DARK BROWN EYES
Bordeaux

DARK BROWN EYES
Bronze/Gold

If You Have Gray Hair

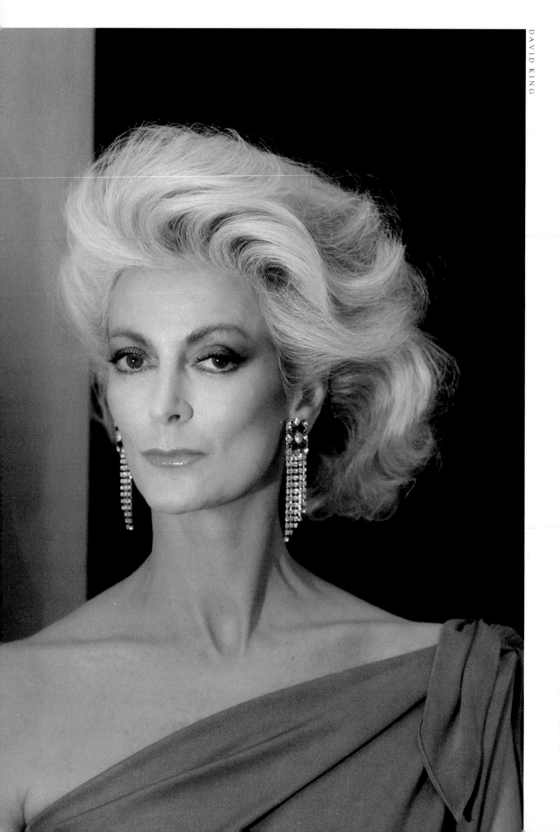

DAVID KING

Carmen is famous because she has gray hair, but she was famous before she had gray hair. Now, though, she looks like a dream, an elegant memory, using smoky pastels to coordinate with the smoky gray of her hair. A siren at any age, but never as much as now.

Foundation Color for Gray Hair

Since the color of your skin doesn't change, check the color chart until you identify your pair of colors and blend. Go darker if you have a tan.

Eye Color for Gray Hair

Stay away from iridescent or frosted shadows! You don't need them; they'll work against the natural shine, texture and natural play of light and shadow your hair already possesses. Go for flat, true colors, the ones you'll find on the chart.

For all gray-haired women, regardless of eye color, the three basic shadows will be coffee, nutmeg/dark beige and mustard yellow. For shadowing or framing, the five option colors are listed on the chart according to your eye color. When buying any of these colors, double check to make sure they're not frosted or iridescent.

Cheek Color for Gray Hair

Never use frosted colors; they accentuate what you want to play down—lines, wrinkles, the elements that age you. Your classic cheek colors are a tawny blush or pure cinnamon. Chestnut is a universal option, as are apricot and soft sienna. For options coordinated with your eye color, just check the chart. Whatever your eye color, you'll be using a bronze blusher to contour.

Lip Color for Gray Hair

No shimmers or metallics on your lips, either! But you can use a bronze or sienna no matter what your eye color. Specific lip colors to complement your eyes appear on your chart.

Gray Hair

Eyes

Coffee

Nutmeg/Dark beige

Mustard yellow

BLUE EYES
Gray mauve

GREEN EYES
Iris

HAZEL EYES
Willow green

BROWN EYES
Terra-cotta

DARK BROWN EYES
Viridian

$\mathscr{C}$heeks

$\mathscr{L}$ips

Tawny blush

Pure cinnamon

Bronze

Sienna

BLUE EYES
Peach rouge

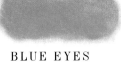

GREEN EYES
Sandalwood rouge

BLUE EYES
Classic peach

GREEN EYES
Soft peach

HAZEL EYES
Soft sienna

BROWN EYES
Pure bronze

HAZEL EYES
Rose peach

BROWN EYES
Classic pink

DARK BROWN EYES
Coco creme

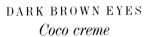

DARK BROWN EYES
Clear red

If You're an Exotic Type

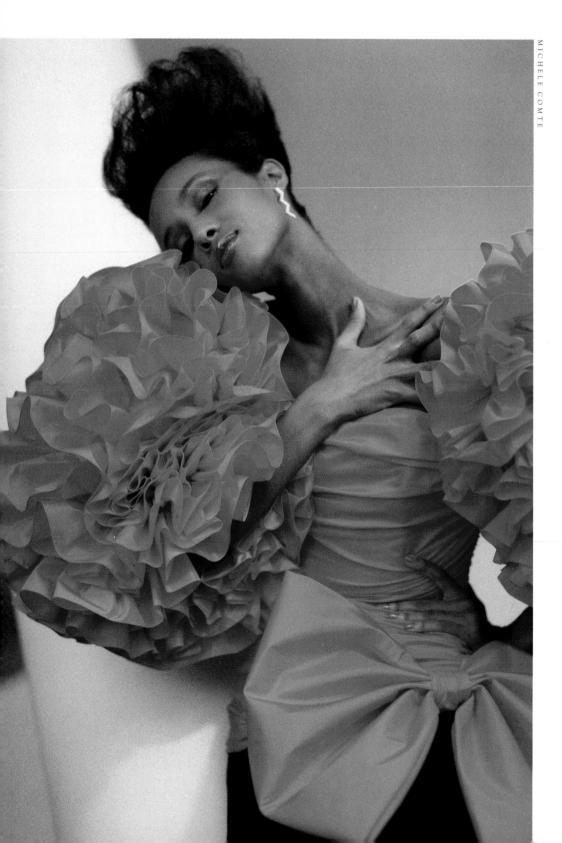

MICHELE COMTE

Iman, milk chocolate to die, whose fine bones and skin tone enable her to model almost anything— fluffy red evening dresses, batik sarongs, you name it, Iman makes it look like art. And that face. She's completely Audrey Hepburn. And so natural! Look again and you'll see that she's completely made up . . . and how you can achieve the same effects, some of the same effects, if your skin is in the same tonal range.

Foundation for Exotics

The "tone" of your skin color is more intense than your paler sisters. I'll go into more detail in Chapter 10, but, to generalize, most Hispanic and Asian skins take medium beige to tawny or deep olive and honey—always blended. Since there is such a broad range of black skin tones, let's look at the foundation chart starting from the fourth grouping down and continuing for three sequences, we're looking at the exotic skin range. Notice what happens. There are two distinctly different tones to the skin tints: The ones on the left have a predominant yellow, the ones on the right, a predominant gray. Chocolate combines them both. I think you'll agree, after a thorough complexion inspection, that your skin tone is predominantly gray or yellow or, maybe, a unique mixture of both. You know what I'd do? I'd play with the samples in the store, mixing them on the back of your wrist before trying the blend on your neck. You may actually have to buy three foundations, but, let me assure you, when you hit it right, when you're applying another layer of your own color to your skin, you feel doubly like yourself— meganatural.

Eye Color for Women Who Are Black, Asian, Hispanic and Olive-Skinned

Here's my basic principle for all exotic types: The darker your skin, the more dramatically colored shadow your eyes can accommodate. You have my permission to go darker and more intense, but that doesn't mean you have to limit yourself to black liner. Exotic skin can take more color. The three basic shadow/liners that will work on Asian, Hispanic and Black skins alike are royal blue, lavender and mahogany. Choices for particular eye colors appear on the chart.

Cheek Color for Exotic Skin Tones

If you're Black, Asian, Hispanic or, in general, have dark olive skin, you're got a more vibrant range of cheek color from which to choose. Your blushers are classic rose, classic tomato or earth red. For shading, you'll be using a dark contour cream no matter what your skin color, and you'll need a highlight cream that comes in a single dark but lighter tone.

Lip Color for Exotic Skin Tones

Here's where you can really afford to make a more dramatic color statement than people with paler skin. Your classic lip colors are bronze/copper, deep sienna orange and matte red. You can play with mahogany, soft plum, burnt orange or red. The perfect lip shade to complement your eyes appears on the chart. No matter what the color of your eyes, you'll find dark contour cream evens out lips.

Exotics

Black

Skin

Eyes

Royal blue

Lavender

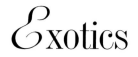

Mahogany

GREEN EYES
Granite

HAZEL EYES
Classic terra-cotta

LIGHT BROWN EYES
Charcoal

DARK BROWN EYES
Blue-gray

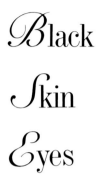

BROWN-BLACK EYES
Deep olive

Exotic Cheeks

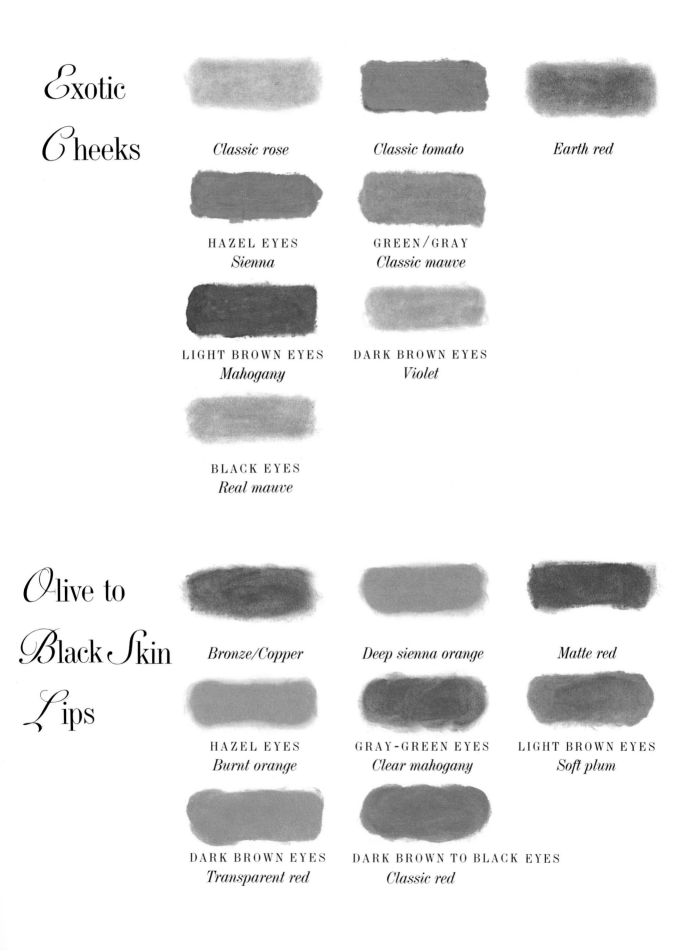

Classic rose

Classic tomato

Earth red

HAZEL EYES
Sienna

GREEN/GRAY
Classic mauve

LIGHT BROWN EYES
Mahogany

DARK BROWN EYES
Violet

BLACK EYES
Real mauve

Olive to Black Skin Lips

Bronze/Copper

Deep sienna orange

Matte red

HAZEL EYES
Burnt orange

GRAY-GREEN EYES
Clear mahogany

LIGHT BROWN EYES
Soft plum

DARK BROWN EYES
Transparent red

DARK BROWN TO BLACK EYES
Classic red

Shimmer Powders

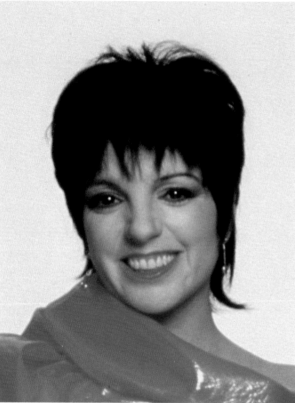

*I*n the case of evening colors, flip to the "Evening Colors" page; there you'll find shimmer powders, to use on eyes, cheeks, lips and collarbones if they're bare. But remember, the shimmer colors you select for evening are always coordinated with what you're wearing, not with hair and eyes. Let's say you're wearing an ice-blue gown. I'd recommend you use a slate gray liner and your blush as eye shadow. Keep the mouth pale. Think about a silvery shimmer powder that will bring out the "ice" in the "ice blue." The point: Don't try to match or overwhelm the gown.

Evening for everybody Here's the great Liza, creating out of her dramatic coloring a consummately dramatic evening look that you simply can't forget. The hair's pastel intense, as are the colors of the eyes, the cheeks, the lips.

Shimmer Powders

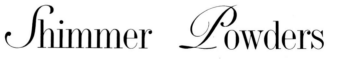

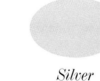

Opalescent   Silver   Gold   Fuchsia

Bronze   Slate   Dark bronze

The Next Step

So that's all there is to using the charts. See how easy it is. Remember, the charts are repeated on perforated pages at the back of the book so you don't have to take the book with you when you shop for makeup.

Now you're ready to combine what you learned about equipment and what you learned about color into the next stage: the art of application.

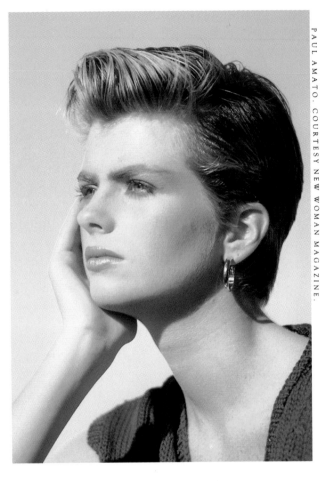

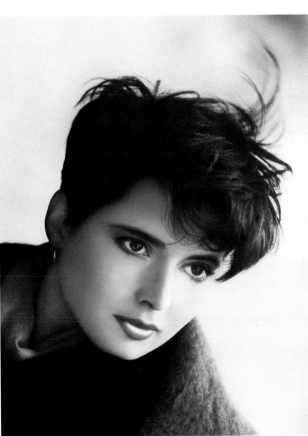

The tones of makeup change the way the seasons do. Winter makeup should have a smudgier, shady feeling to the eyes and more definition to the cheeks and lips, as you see on Isabella. The reason: You're wearing more layers of clothing in heavier fabrics and often darker colors, which means your face needs more emphasis. Summer makeup, shown here on Deirdre McGuire, should be peachier, sunnier, and be more naturally blended to skin tone, since you're showing more of it and because fabrics and colors are lighter.

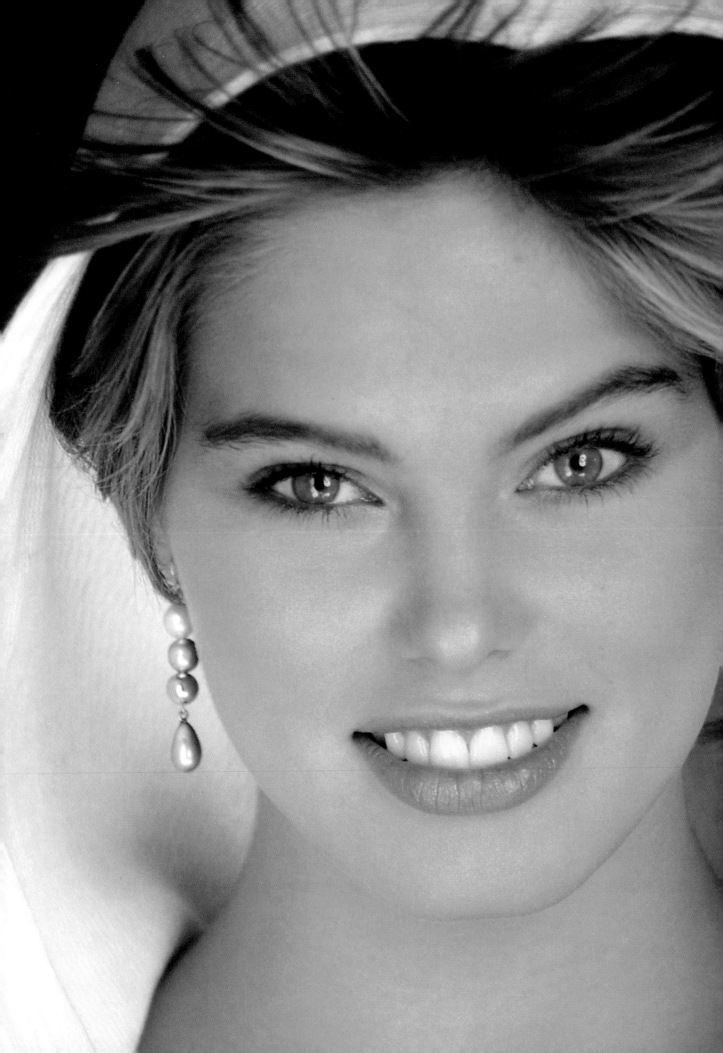

Part Two

The Beauty Part

———

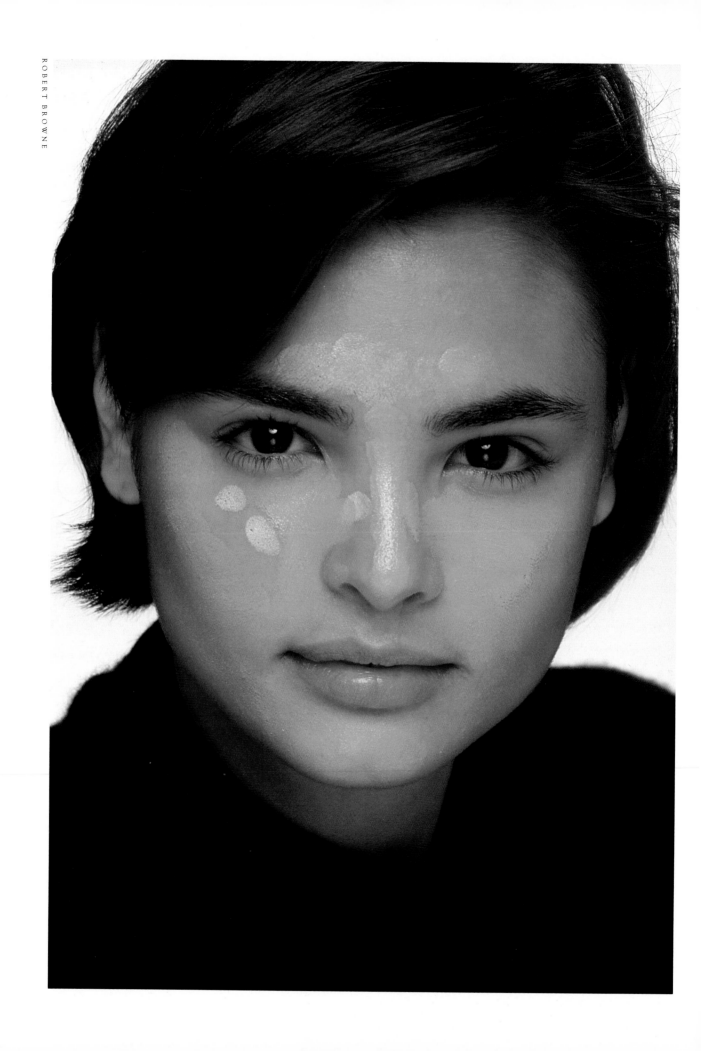

3

Preparing the Canvas of Your Face

To touch, to kiss, to caress—these are the desires you want to encourage. And they revolve around the mystique of soft, dewy skin. Since we "encounter" people primarily with our faces, our facial skin should suggest natural, healthy, all-over touchability. Skin that glows like silk—that's "the skin you love to touch." A smooth, even skin tone that reflects serenity and refinement is at the heart of New Classic Beauty—and here's how to achieve it. Don't worry if there are flaws. They can always be corrected.

Priming Your Face

Properly preparing your face to "accept" foundation can make a crucial difference in your finished look. First, wash your face thoroughly with whatever preparation is recommended for your skin type—cleansing cream for dry skin, a liquid cleanser for oily skin then rinsed with clear, tepid water. (By the way, one of the benefits of New Classic Beauty is that it stays on all day, which means that it stays on, period, so you have to take

Talisa Soto
The prettiest skin in town
—in progress

some care when you wash to make sure no vestige of makeup remains.)

Remember, you can't overrinse your face. Still the most perfect liquid, water will refresh as it cleans. I tell my clients to stand before the basin and splash repeatedly, even if the floor gets wet, then gently towel dry. (A tip: If you're taking a long, skin-drying airplane trip, flush your face frequently with water; it'll keep it from drying out.)

Once your face is clean and dry, you'll be adding moisturizer, also geared to skin type. I'm assuming that, as a sophisticated cosmetics user, you have devoted time and money to finding the right moisturizer for your skin type, so I'm going to skip the basics and concentrate on a few points that are crucial.

- Steer clear of perfumed moisturizers. The more scent in the product, the greater its chances of irritating your skin. My personal favorite is any product containing aloe. Whether you're on the beach or in an overheated winter apartment, aloe vera gives moisture and glow. I wouldn't be without it. Don't you!

- Moisturizer should never be massaged into the skin; it should be lightly layered with the fingertips and allowed to be absorbed.
- Every woman should use plenty of moisturizer, regardless of age or skin type, because skin that is moisturized "takes" makeup more easily. If your skin is plumped up, cosmetics will go on smoother, sheerer and not get "stuck" in lines.
- Make sure your moisturizer has been absorbed completely before applying foundation! If you follow this rule, you can be confident your makeup won't run. *Don't rush this vital step!* If your moisturizer has been thoughtfully and carefully applied and given enough time to be absorbed by your skin, no excess film will remain. Your skin will simply feel soft and silky smooth.

Now that you've cleansed and moisturized, you're almost ready to apply your foundation. But first, one important step: the complexion inspection.

The Complexion Inspection

*I*t's amazing how successfully facial blemishes can be camouflaged if you know where the "trouble" areas are. Take a cold, hard look at your cleansed and dried face before doing anything else. Don't panic over a blemish or a red spot. Use an undertoner instead. I'll be discussing undertoner in more detail later, but for now remember to use

undertoner only on problem areas; it is a cover-all only in one special case, which you'll read about. If your skin is generally clear, but you notice trouble around the eyes and nose, or if your laugh lines seem obvious, you'll work with cover creams, highlighters, pencils and light foundations that give the illusion of smooth and dewy skin.

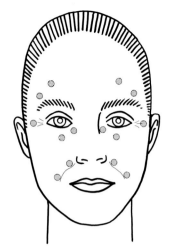

The white dots on Phoebe Cates's face are moisturizer applied extra heavily in the areas where skin is driest. If your skin is dry, try using two coats of moisturizer; it'll make your skin positively dewy. Just make sure it's completely absorbed before you apply base.

Cover-up Creams and Undertoners

These marvelously effective products, applied with a cover-up brush, are used to make valleys, blemishes and laugh lines vanish. Here's what you should use:

- For extra fair skin, use *green undertoner.*
- For all other skins, including exotics, use *turquoise cover-up cream.*
- For birthmarks or scars, use *aqua undertoner.*

- If you're pale, you've been in the sun too much and have developed a leathery look to your skin, *always use an undertoner over your complete face* after applying moisturizer and before foundation.
- To cover dark circles and laugh lines, use a pale *undereye cover cream* if your skin is light to medium and a darker shade if your skin is in the medium-olive-to-black range.

Remember, the purpose of foundation is to enhance, not announce! So if you're careless in applying and choosing the color of your foundation, there'll be a line of demarcation at

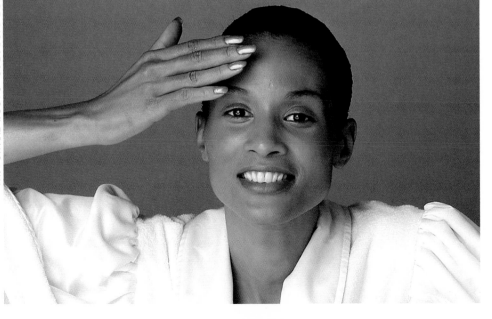

The lovely Beverly Johnson never looking happier while applying moisturizer. The lesson of these pictures is that putting on makeup should be a sensual experience, and nothing, I mean *nothing,* feels as soothing as good moisturizer marrying with your pores. It feels fabulous!

the jawline—a dead giveaway that you've got something to hide. When you're dealing with exotic skin, always remember: There are two basic tones in dark skins, one predominantly gray, one predominantly yellow. With the proper turquoise undertoner and the right makeup, which you're here to learn, you can turn gray to a beautiful sable-silver mahogany and the yellow to burnished, rich toasted golden brown. If you're Hispanic or Asian, you'll want to use a green undertoner to erase the sallowness and then use some tawny foundation to burnish the skin.

The object of foundation color is to give the impression of no makeup at all; you must always remember that, it's basic to the New Classic look. I've mentioned a little about foundation in Chapter 2, but here's my lecture on the essentials of using foundation correctly:

The Terrific Ten

*T*here are about ten basic foundation colors, ranging from pure ivory to chocolate. Divided into pairs according to the intensity of your skin tone, they can be combined to provide the right tint for any individual skin. The pairs are: (1) light skin will take bases from pure ivory to the beige, most Occidental skins take light beige to medium beige; (2) most Occidental skins with an olive tint take medium beige to tawny tan; (3) light Exotic takes deep olive to toasted honey; (4) medium Exotic takes desert tan and (5) the darkest skin takes mahogany (if gray tinted) and chocolate (if yellow tinted). Ebony is for the very darkest skin tone. In addition to being universally useful, these colors have another thing in common: *They contain no red.*

You want foundation without a lot of color, most particularly the color red, because you're trying to duplicate your natural skin tone, specifically the color of the skin on your neck. Remember, foundation should never *add* color; rouge or blusher does that. It should only *soften*, *smooth* and *refine*, or camouflage pimples, birthmarks, scars, undereye bags, laugh lines and crow's-feet.

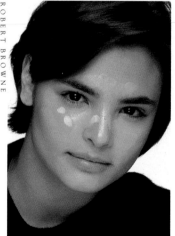

Ykkk! Talisa Soto has blue dots on her face! Is this a horror movie? *Au contraire,* it's a beauty lesson because those blue dots are a combination of moisturizer and undertoner, blended to soften her skin so that it will "take" the eye, cheek and skin makeup.

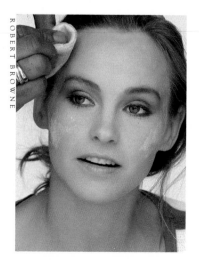

You can see from this shot of Lisa Ryall where foundation should go and how it's blended with a sponge. If your skin is clear, you have no reason to use base all over your face. Concentrate on the places where more makeup is going to be applied.

How to Choose the Right Color for You

*M*ost white and olive skin tones rarely match with a single base color, but are instead within the range of the two colors suggested. Therefore, a single foundation can make your face appear pasty and masklike, as if there was a ring around your face. If you blend your bases you'll bring out the highlights of your natural skin tones.

From the foundation chart, pick the two colors listed as being in your natural range, then, using your neck tone as a guide, blend the two colors on a white piece of paper or in your hand until the result is a perfect match. All skin has both light and dark hues; if you've blended the two bases well and applied them correctly, the contrasting play of light and shadow will be beautifully enhanced.

Where Does the Color Go?

*T*he color of your face before makeup is essentially the same as after. What you're really doing is enhancing your complexion, and the highlights and shadows of your facial planes, with undertones, highlighters and contouring. To achieve those ends, you'll basically be keeping the center of your face *light* while *framing* it with blusher and contouring rouge.

I define "center," or the "light area," as from your forehead, under your eyes and down the center of your nose to the top lip. You're always striving for highlight and contour, light and dark, so everything—from undertoner to foundations—should be blended, never rubbed in. You're not attempting to *change* the color of your skin; you're trying to accentuate it. If your face doesn't look natural, you're not making it up, you're painting it! With practice, you'll learn to mix and blend various foundations (see my color charts for the tones you can play with according to the color of your skin, hair and eyes). Dot the blended foundation on your face, then smooth it gently with a damp silk sponge for maximum sheerness.

Translucent Powder

*D*on't be afraid of looking pasty. Applied lightly and thoroughly dusted off with a powder brush, this wonderful substance sets your makeup and inhibits shine. Translucent powder doesn't add color, and can be used on most skin tones, including Black, Hispanic and Asian. If, after dusting off, translucent powder shows white against darker skin, try a tinted shade, but always try translucent first. Since it's colorless, you won't risk altering the tone of your base.

Special Skin Problems

Touching

Women tend to rub their skin, especially during stressful periods, usually without even being aware of it. *Stop doing it!* Even resting your chin in your hands can deposit dirt and oil in the skin, and that can lead to breakouts and acne. Make yourself aware of this habit and give it up!

Freckles

Although they're cute as a button on a six-year-old, freckles tend to lose their charm as we age. And they are the first sign of your skin's intolerance for the sun! The best way to avoid or downplay freckling is to avoid the sun, but if you won't, always use a heavy sunscreen block either under your moisturizer or one that contains it. Even indoors and in town, always be sure to use a sunscreen!

Sensitive Skin

It used to be thought that delicate, allergy-prone skin was a problem of fair women exclusively. Now we know differently. Sensitive skin causes many different reactions, from a tendency to drying and chafing to breakouts, hives and blotching. If you have sensitive skin, be sure to avoid heavily perfumed products and use only the mildest and detergent-free cosmetics. Wash your face no more than twice a day, avoid scrubs and toners and use a soft towel to *blot*—not rub—your skin dry. For you, too, avoiding the sun, or making sure you never go to the beach without a heavy sunscreen block and a hat, is a necessity!

Large Pores

Commonly associated with oily skin, this condition is chronic. Frankly, there's not much permanent correction for this, but there are some very effective cosmetic ways of temporarily making pores seem smaller. Using an astringent toner or exfoliating lotion not only cleanses and refreshes oily skin, it also "plumps up" skin, giving the impression of smaller pores. There are also specific foundations, usually powder-based, that are designed to minimize large pores, and a translucent powder as a "finisher" will do wonders to produce the illusion of more delicate skin.

Acne Scars

If pitting and scarring is not severe, hypoallergenic cover-up foundations can make an enormous difference. For more severe conditions, you might want to try dermabrasion, or injections of silicone or collagen to plump up depressions and produce a smoother skin surface. See a dermatologist who is best qualified to advise you on a course of action. Remember, collagen face creams are not miracle creams because, as a topical agent, the substance doesn't work for more than a couple of hours. If you're interested in collagen, you'll have to consider surgical injection.

The State of the Art

Now that the canvas of your face is properly primed, and your skin is ultrareceptive, we turn to styling your features—eyes, cheeks and lips—so they show your true colors: vibrant, glowing and wonderfully refined.

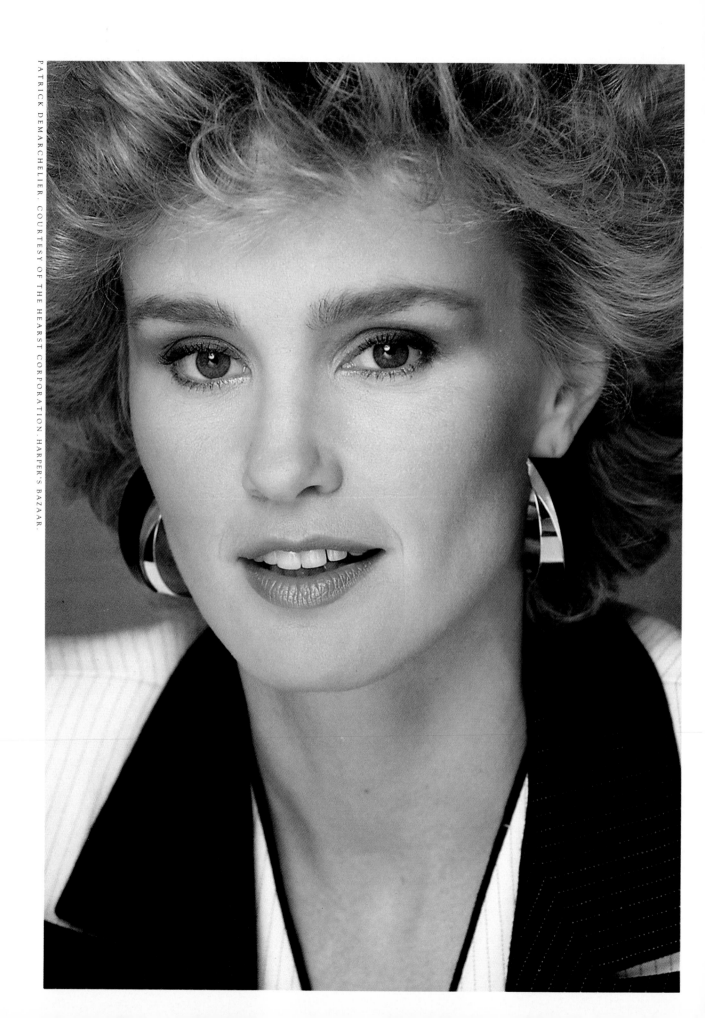

4

The Eyes Have It

Eyes: The Windows of the Soul

Look someone directly in the eye, and you immediately learn a lot about them. Nothing is as pleasing as a direct gaze because it shows you have nothing to hide, that you're confident of what you are. To me, as a makeup artist, the eyes are the focal point of the face, the absolute center of attention for the same reason: They're the most immediate channel of your essential self, the means of announcing you're naturally glamorous and not too timid to show it.

I've come to realize that what is really responsible for the dramatic power of the eyes isn't color, it's shape! Shaping the eye is what my makeup is all about, the shape and the softness of color that is the key to a natural-looking yet sophisticated makeup. You should never be struck by the vibrancy of a woman's eye shadow. There should never be color jumping out at you. Subtlety is the essence, for night and day, subtlety that will always make you look alert, attractive—and young for your age.

Jessica Lange
The hypnotic allure of
beautiful eyes

The New Classic Beauty Mistake-Proof System for Perfectly Gorgeous Eyes

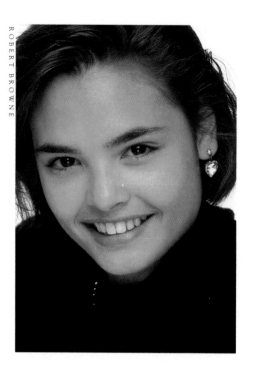

In this before and after sequence, look for this: before, she's cute, but there's a strong downward pull to her features because the eyes are the smallest, therefore the weakest, feature on the face. By subtly opening the eyes and adding the slightest bit of blusher to throw attention upward, I've realigned her whole face so the features are balanced.

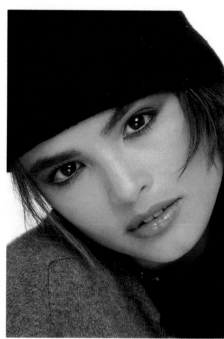

*O*nce you've mastered these easy, basic steps, you'll never have trouble applying eye makeup again. Just follow these instructions precisely; believe me, they work!

• First, make sure your lids are free of oil or excess moisturizer; if they're not, they won't "hold" color, which will tend to fade or crease or smudge off. For extra protection, dab a little transparent powder over lids, then dust off excess with a cotton ball or your cleanup brush.

• Next, choose two eye shadows, one darker and one lighter, from the color chart, according to your skin, hair and eye tones—your personal color scheme.

• Begin with the lighter shadow, which will almost always be in caramel, cinnamon, terra-cotta or a pale gray or desert gold. With a small rubber blending sponge, apply shadow. Start at the base of your lashes, sweep up and above it to the brow.

• Take up the darker shadow—perhaps

Caution: All illustrations represent makeup before blending.

brown, teal, smoky colors, mauve, olive, russet, burgundy or coffee, depending on your coloring—and apply it from the center of your eyelid along (and above) the crease out toward the temple, creating an almond shape (how high depends on the shape and size of your eyes and your face). To add some extra oomph, you may want to apply a highlighter (coordinated to the other two shadows) over the brow bone.

Using the sponge applicator, blend the line of demarcation between the colors until they become seamless.

- Now you're ready to line your eyes. With a moistened liner brush, apply a dark shadow to the top eyelid, directly above the lashes, then below the lower lashes in a very thin, very narrow line. The color should be dark, but black or really vibrant colors should be used only by brunettes or women with exotic looks. If you don't exercise extreme caution with heavy effects, you're going to find yourself looking more exotic than you intended!

- If you've always thought that lining your eyes was beyond you, you'll be amazed at how easy it is. Here's a tip for finishing liner to ensure a slightly softened but still well-defined eye that won't fade or smudge in the course of a day. Line eyes with a wet brush then dry the brush with a tissue. Run it through shadow and go over the line you've already made, gently smudge with a cotton swab to soften.

- Brows come next, so take your eyebrow brush and, sweeping upward, form your brows into their maximum natural arch. With a soft pencil, fill in the sparse patches by drawing single imitation hairs, not a strong, solid line. Remember, nothing looks worse than an overtweezed or artificially arched brow. Be sure to

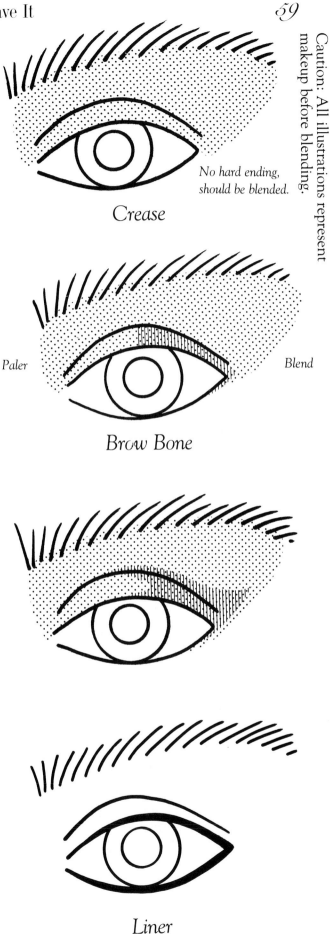

No hard ending, should be blended.

Crease

Paler　　　*Blend*

Brow Bone

Liner

choose an eyebrow pencil that's either the same tone or a bit darker than your natural color; avoid black at all costs!

• Before applying mascara—I prefer charcoal or navy—be sure to use your eyelash curler. Gently grip your lashes and hold for about five seconds. Next, carefully sweep mascara through your upper lashes—twice. Allow ten seconds without blinking between applications so the mascara will set; if you can do this, your mascara will not smear or smudge all day. Once the lashes dry, comb through them with the eyelash comb to remove any clumpy, excess mascara. Unless your lashes are blond, you should never use mascara on the lower lashes. Framing the eye with shadow liner gives you all the accentuation you'll need.

A special note about mascara: As I said, I don't recommend using mascara on the bottom lashes unless they are blond; there are, however, two exceptions: blue eyes, when the second coat of mascara can be navy, applied to both top and bottom lashes; and brown or hazel eyes, when you'll recoat lashes with mascara that's dark green or mauve, respectively. You won't believe how this enhances the sparkle and vibrancy of your eyes!

• If your lashes are unusually sparse or if you really want your eyes to look lush, apply a false eyelash or two. They come in strips but are applied one by one. Grip lash with a tweezer, dip in transparent glue and simply place where you want it to go.

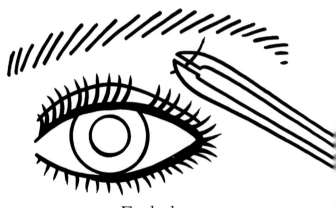

Eyelashes

Special Advice for Special Cases

If Your Eyes Are Close-set

You want to emphasize the outer corners of the lid. Apply the lighter shadow from the center of the eye to the nose. Next, sweep the darker shadow from the center of the eye out toward the temple, then blend together the two colors with a sponge applicator.

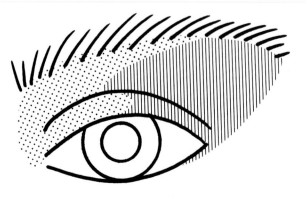

Close-Set Eyes

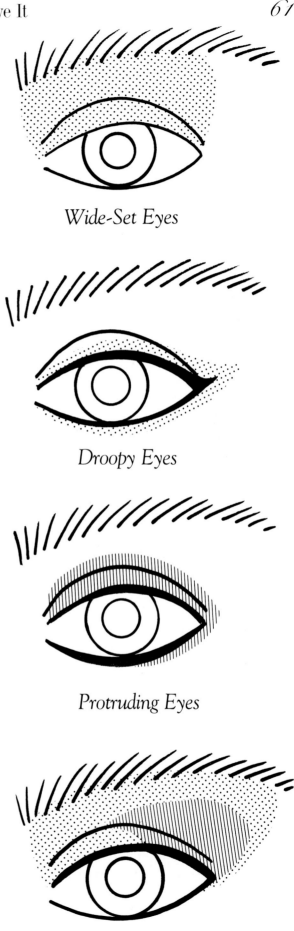

If Your Eyes Are Wide-set

Start shadows at the eye's inner corner, but do not extend them beyond the outer corner.

Wide-Set Eyes

If Your Eyes Droop

Use liner along the lashes but bring it up slightly at the outer corners. Blend eye shadow with a dry brush over the line to soften it.

Droopy Eyes

If Your Eyes Protrude

Use darker shadow over the lid and crease, then intensify liner along the bottom lashes to provide the illusion that your eyes recede. Frosted shadows are not for you; stick to matte products.

Protruding Eyes

If Your Eyes Are Deep-set

First, line your upper lashes, then, starting in the middle of the crease, blend darker shadow outward to the corner. Apply lighter color from the lashes to the base of the brow. You may want to carry the darker shading higher, even all the way into the brow, so that when your eyes are open, some blending of tone is evident, causing the eye to "pop." Be sure to line your eyes; it'll also help bring deep-set eyes to the fore!

Deep-Set Eyes

If Your Face Is Narrow

To give your face a more oval appearance, carry your darker eye shadow farther toward your temples, parallel with the upper sweep of your rouge. Your lighter shadow will go from the crease to the brow and extend over the hairline, above the rouge. If you use the proper soft colors and blend rouge and shadows well, you'll be amazed at how much more oval your face becomes.

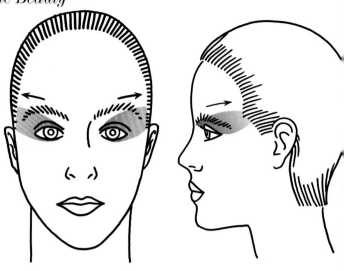

Narrow Face

If Your Face Is Wide

Eye color should never extend all the way out to the temple, and darker shadow should be used on the inner corners.

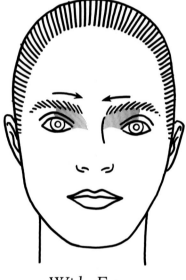

Wide Face

If You Wear Glasses

Whether you wear specs all the time, some of the time or occasionally as a "kicky" fashion accessory, you'll be thrilled with these special tips.

All the Time

You must wear strong eye makeup. Wearing glasses "dims" eye makeup, so your eyes are going to need a bit more strength and intensity while making sure you don't overdo it. Just how strong you decide to do your eyes depends on the darkness of your lenses; the darker the lens, the more intense the makeup.

Eyebrows are superimportant when you wear glasses. Eyeglass frames throw extra emphasis on the brows, so here's some good advice for impeccable brow grooming: Before you go to sleep, apply a nonoily night cream with an eyebrow brush into the hairs, brush upward creating as much of a natural arch as your brows will allow. You'll see very quickly how successfully brows can be trained to look their best.

Here is a list of the ways you can intensify eye makeup while maintaining the new classic look:

- Frame your eyes in color. For example, while continuing to use elegant "neutrals" as your dark and light shadows, you can go with a blue liner. Although very dark liners—brown, charcoal or slate—are preferred for the naked eye, the bespectacled one will look great with a more vibrant liner tone. Just make sure it's not too heavy and that it's properly softened with a dried brush and shadow after the first application.

- When you wear glasses, you've got to downplay mascara. If your lenses are thick, they'll literally magnify your eyes and lashes, so don't overdo it. Remember to comb through your lashes after each of your two applications, and never use mascara on the bottom ones. If you are very fair, you might want to have your lashes dyed, but don't try to do it yourself. Always consult a professional.

Some of the Time

- If you use glasses only for reading, apply your makeup as if you don't wear glasses at all. That's because women who wear glasses primarily for reading usually take them off when they greet or talk to people. For all practical makeup and social purposes, you don't wear glasses.

- As a fashion accessory: Treat your frames as you would any other accessory, don't let it clash. For instance, dark red lip color with fuchsia frames is a major mistake, as are peach frames with burgundy lips. You must always coordinate frame and makeup, but never, never match them, and remember, glasses make a very strong statement, so you must appropriately tone down lips, shadow and rouge to accommodate them.

Don't ever pick eyeglass frames to go with your clothes, but always coordinate them with your skin, hair and eye colors. To make sure you achieve the right coordination, use my color charts. They'll even help you choose the most flattering frame. Coordinate them the

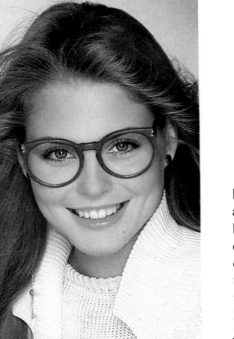

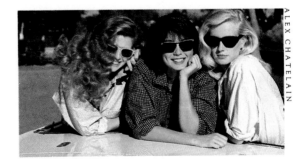

Does this girl look adorable or what! Notice how the red frames coordinate with her lip color and rouge, and how the size of the lenses and the tint make the beautiful blue of her eyes just bounce. Don't tell *me* eyeglasses aren't an accessory!

I've included this second picture because I love it. And because I love dark glasses. Dramatic effect —to be used only when you're making it part of your impression. And always in L.A.

*L*isa *R*yall

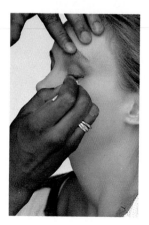

ROBERT BROWNE

Pay attention to this sequence of photos of me doing Lisa's eyes. For instance, see how I'm extending her brow with the pencil, the way I've extended her eye makeup toward the temple. The combination makes the eyes look larger and more shapely.

You would never know from looking at Lisa's eyes that she's actually wearing three colors of eye shadow because they're so blended. When you're making up, don't stop until you can only see a single color.

The colors I'm using to shadow and to line her eyes aren't actually *colors*; they're earth tones. Her eyes, her peachy skin, her naturally tinted lips have enough color. What you want is to enhance the size and shape of the eye, not merely call attention.

Look at me doing a "smudge" on Lisa's lower lid. Lining your eyes doesn't mean the world sees a hard-edged line. It sees what looks like the shadow cast by thick bottom lashes. So underlining is a form of eye shadow too; that's why I recommend using dry shadow powder applied with a wet brush. It smudges more easily.

As I apply her mascara, I'm actually lifting the skin of her eye crease upward, pulling the lashes away from the eye. This'll guarantee you neat application every time.

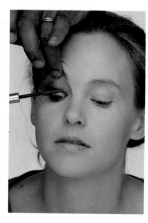
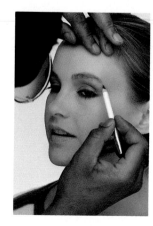
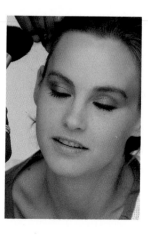

way you coordinate blush and lip pencil; they're another accessory, not a major attraction. You probably guessed, I love neutral color frames from tawny tortoise to thin gold wire.

• Tinted lenses: Here, too, more intense makeup is required because colored lenses soften all tones. This is one of the rare cases in which you might want to consider using black liner and shadow that's almost "evening" in intensity. Not frosts or metallics, but slate or a dark blue-gray, always well blended and carefully applied. Cheek color, too, should have a more than daytime vibrancy.

If You Wear Contact Lenses

As most lens wearers know from experience, mascara can be a real problem. A single flake drifting into the eye can cause redness and tearing. Here are a few hints to save you anguish and embarrassment:

• You're best off with a mascara devised for sensitive skin, but, in any case, stay away from lash-lengtheners because their tiny fibers are an invitation to disaster. Make sure you comb your lashes thoroughly after applying mascara to make sure no stray flakes are left to cause trouble. And you might want to start your mascara a small distance from the lash base.

• The New Classic Beauty System is actually great for you, since experts recommend that lens wearers choose powdered shadows and steer away from liquid eyeliners. Stay away from frosted shadows, too, which may contain irritating metallic particles.

• Be sure to use an oil-free makeup remover, since oil can seep into the eye.

• Wearing the new colored contacts can be lots of fun; it's experimental, it's different and it can be startling without being shocking. It also gives you a good excuse to play around with a wide range of different makeup colors, which you can choose from the color charts.

Why Eye Makeup Is Major Magic

*Y*ou've got great-looking eyes now, the kind of understated yet dramatic eyes that men—and women—rarely turn away from. They radiate everything you want to project about yourself: a strong and calm self-image, a free and open enjoyment of life and a marvelously flattering ability to look at people and show them you're really listening to them. That's charm, and it's yours.

This is how strongly I feel about eye makeup. Once you master the basic techniques, you can get away with wearing almost no other cosmetics except lip color and moisturizer. The only thing people will notice is that you never looked better!

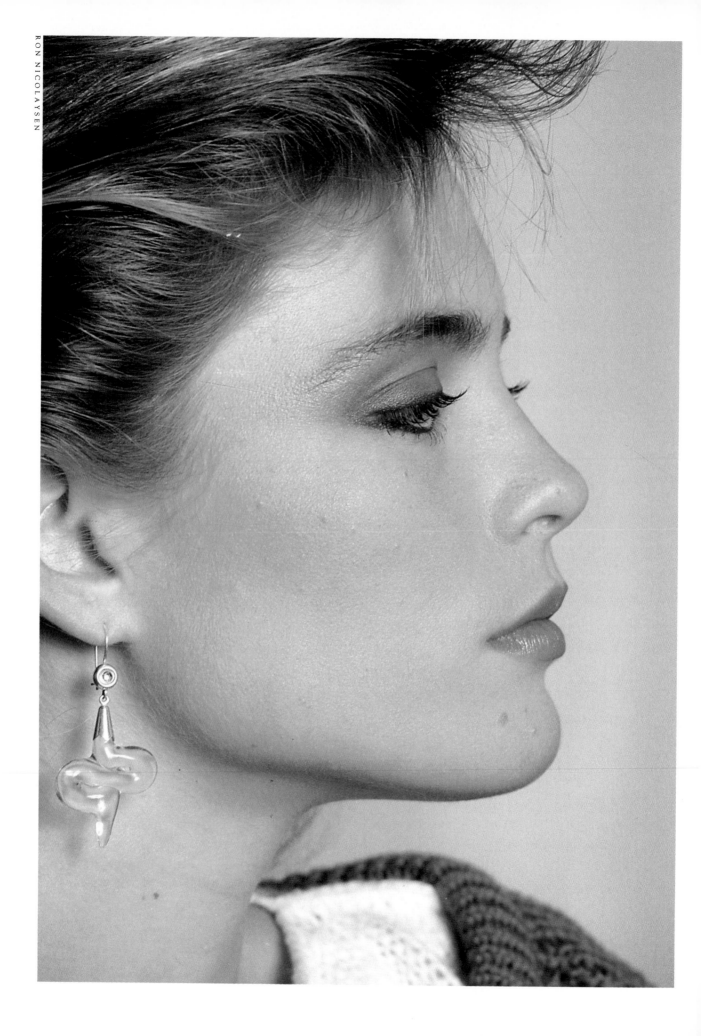

5

Cheek to Cheek—
Designing Your Bone Structure

Makeup Miracles—Guaranteed!

*Y*ou're about to become a magician. Don't be shocked. It's true! But you're not going to change rabbits into flowers or make nickels appear from behind somebody's ear. No, you're going to perform a far more amazing trick: You're going to change the shape of your face. Whether God gave you a wider face than you'd have liked, or a narrower one; whether you'd have preferred Garbo's cheekbones to your own; if you can't seem to do anything about the slight beginnings of a double chin—it doesn't matter, because you're going to transform your face into the shape and bone structure you've always dreamed of. Sound impossible? Believe me, it isn't. Not only is it possible, it's not even difficult. Trust me, once you master my techniques of shading and contouring, you'll have the face you've always wanted!

Kim Alexis
Shaping perfection

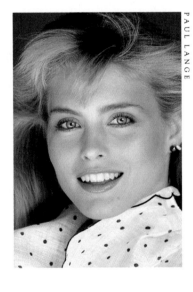

Is there anything wrong with Kim Alexis's face? No, not really, but you can see from this shot that from some angles her face has a real squareness. What I did about that was apply blusher almost laterally, from the mideye outward, then take it up.

Remember what I told you about highlighting the center of the face. In Kim's case, the marvelous features were emphasized, and the contouring is aligned with the eyes so that you really don't notice the shape of the face.

The Beautiful Oval

*E*veryone wants the perfect face: big doe-eyes, naturally high cheekbones, a slightly rounded square jaw, a long neck, high forehead and an oval countenance. That's because any woman given the chance to look like Audrey Hepburn or Grace Kelly would go for it. Unfortunately, the Hepburn/Kelly level of beauty is very rare. Still, with my New Classic Beauty, you can come a lot closer to the ideal than you ever thought possible, whether your face is round, rectangular or square!

What really matters, for all face shapes, is balance and composition. The "oval" has come to be considered the classic shape. So I'm going to show how, by the application of color on your particular face shape, you can create the marvelous illusion of the perfect oval. The process is called "face shaping," and it refers to applying color to your face to contour, and add shape—without sacrificing the skin's natural hue.

Show and Tell

I always insist that my private clients begin their face shaping lessons with an examination of their bones, especially their cheekbones. Simply place your hands on your face, feel your forehead, work your way down the sides of your face, feeling the cheekbones down to the chin, then across the jawline. Color should go *over* the bones—a bit on the cheekbones, on either side of the forehead, a touch on the chin. That's the recipe for perfect balance, enhancing the look of symmetry for which we all starve.

How to Look Simply Peachy!

*O*ne of the guiding principles of New Classic Beauty is that no matter what your own coloring, you want to strive for a warm, peachy glow. You'll achieve this with two colors of blush, chosen from the blush color chart, one dark (for contouring or face shaping) and one light (for color). You'll apply and blend them as follows:

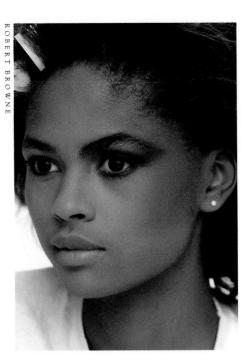

ROBERT BROWNE

With your shading brush, apply the darker color, which will be in the cinnamony to taupy range, to and slightly under the cheekbone and along the perimeter of your face up toward the brow line in a pork chop shape. Then, using the color brush, apply the lighter shade directly over the dark, blending them together.

Most women can select the lighter color from peach to coral or pink, but those with darker or olive skin should stick to red, burgundy and mahogany, always applied with a soft touch of flawless blending.

My most important secret to applying cheek color is where the color goes—something many women have had trouble mastering, until now.

Notice the "pork chop" shape of Karen Alexander's rouge. Literally, pork chop. See how it sweeps up to meet her shadow, giving a whole lift to her face? Her blusher actually has a lot of vibrancy, but it's applied ever so lightly and doesn't look overstated.

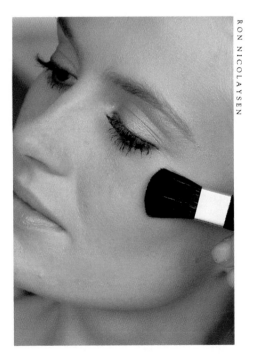

RON NICOLAYSEN

See where that brush is? Don't go any farther toward the nose than that. That is the beginning of the pork chop!

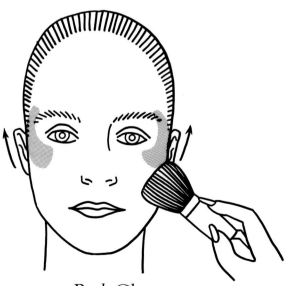

Pork Chops

Cheek color should begin below the center of the eye, at its widest point, then sweep up and around and narrow toward the temple —always *in the shape of a pork chop.* It should extend clear to the brow line until it almost blends with your shadow, but with no hard lines.

Make sure you never put cheek color too close to the nose or too low on the cheeks, where it will actually drag the face down, especially if applied too enthusiastically.

After applying the two rouges, apply a bit of transparent powder with a puff, then brush off the excess with a stroking motion (with the powder brush) and blend out the color slightly.

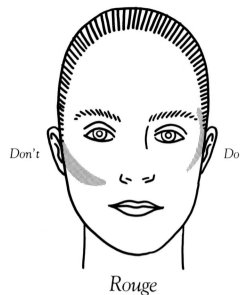

Don't   *Do*

Rouge

Some Other Priceless Cheek Tips I've Collected

*A*fter you've rouged and powdered, stand back and examine your work. Is the color soft, subtle and even? Did you use a light hand? And did you work near a natural light source? If you didn't, how you look in daylight could be an unpleasant surprise!

• Always make it a point to choose cheek color that is close to your own skin tone. The last thing you want is two circles of red in the middle of your face! The goal of face-shaping is to brighten skin and add a blush, not a wallop, of coloring— you'll also be wearing eye makeup and lip color, and it all has to work as a whole. As I've said, the eyes are the centerpiece of the beautiful face, and you don't want to work against that by overemphasizing your cheeks. Strive for cheekbones that are "there" but aren't insisting you notice them!

• It wouldn't hurt to have a friend take a Polaroid of you—before and after applying makeup. You'll be surprised by how much you learn about your face and your makeup skills!

• To balance face color, you might want to add just a tad of your lighter rouge on either side of the base of the nose, where you may have some natural "darkness"; then, still using the contouring brush, apply a slight hint of the same color under the tip of your nose for symmetry. Next, puff translucent powder down the center of your nose and dust it off with the powder brush for a classic, finished

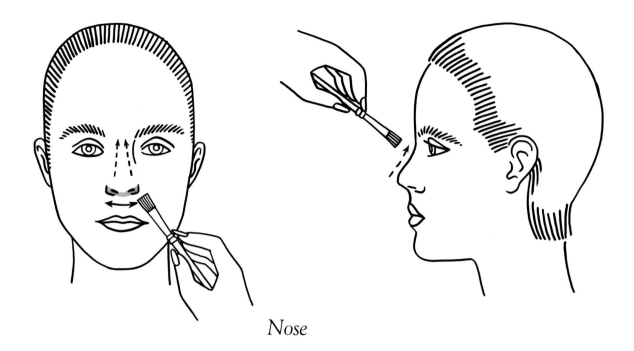

Nose

look. Finally, add the slightest amount of color around the chin and on either side of your forehead with the color brush, brushing it up into the hairline.

· My basic rule for cream versus powder rouge is this: When you're wearing foundation and want a "finished look,"

use the powder. When you want a more natural, healthy glow, use cream over moisturizer followed by translucent powder.

Basically, that's all there is to it, but here's what to do for special cases.

Face Fixes

If Your Face Is Round

What you can't do is "slim" with a dark, smudging contour along the cheekbones; you'll look like someone with a round, dirty face. What you can do is choose cheek colors that have no red, pink, fuchsia or bright tones to them. Gravitate to colors that are "spicy" and have a bit of brown in them, but make sure they're "soft."

Starting with your darker color on your contouring brush, apply from the temple and

go around the end of your eyebrow right out to the hairline and carry it down toward the cheek. *Stop at the top of your cheekbone*—in the pork chop shape. Then, apply the peachier, warmer tone directly over the dark one, but go a little higher, blending with your color brush until the two shades become one. If you've overdone the color, calm it down with some translucent powder.

Brush your darker powder along the jaw-line and below it on both sides of the chin with your slimming brush. After you've brushed

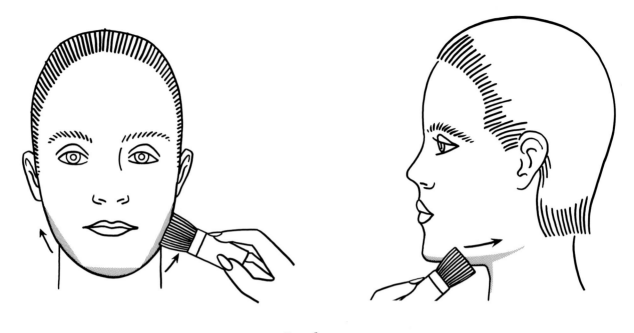

Jawline

color below the chin and blended it well, you'll be amazed at how a double chin seems miraculously to have disappeared! Just make sure your blusher has no red in it; to shadow best, corrective shading and contouring should always be executed with colors from the taupe family.

If Your Face Is Square

Don't use any color blush on the forehead at all and make sure the blushers you choose contain no red or pink. Choose, instead, from the cinnamons and taupes, from colors that are "barely there." You might want to consider eliminating blush altogether and achieving color through a tawny or a peach foundation —one that's slightly darker than your skin tone. The goal is to "smooth over" your natural squareness, and the method you select to achieve that depends on how pale your skin is; the paler the tone, the more you should lean toward foundation alone as a means to achieving the color you want.

To camouflage a double chin: Here's my technique for defining the jawline and making a full chin appear slimmer and squarer: With your slimming brush, very lightly brush contouring rouge under the tip of the chin and along the underedge of the jawbone. By projecting your face away from your neck, you'll turn your chin fleshiness into the illusion of shadow.

If Your Face Is Long and/or Narrow

Keep contouring powder to the perimeter of your face. Sweep it high toward the brow line with your slimming brush, where it should meet and blend with eye shadow (which you extend outward). Select something in the taupy range based on your hair and eye tones. (Stay away from bright color blushes. They'll create too extreme a contrast between the top and bottom half of your face and accentuate the negatives.) The color should look as natural as possible but, by enhancing your upper bone structure (and by highlighting the eyes), direct attention to your face from the bridge of the nose upward. A lip tip: Don't ever use bright or dark lip color! It'll undo all the good I just taught you!

Done perfectly, the use of color and shadowing, of "face shaping" can make a phenomenal contribution to correcting structural facial flaws that have always bugged you. You'll be amazed at the change in yourself, and so will the people who tell you how much thinner you look!

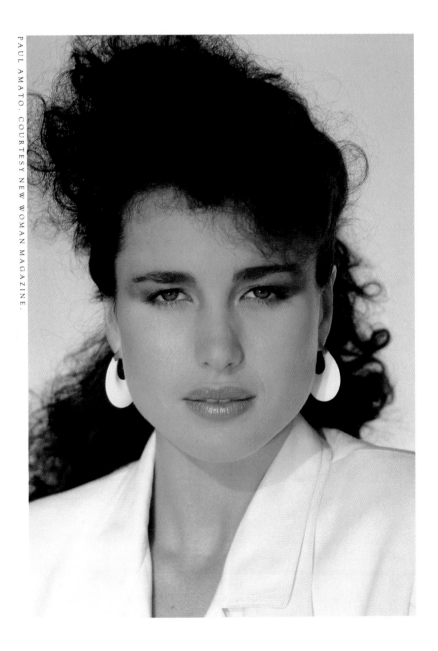

PAUL AMATO. COURTESY NEW WOMAN MAGAZINE.

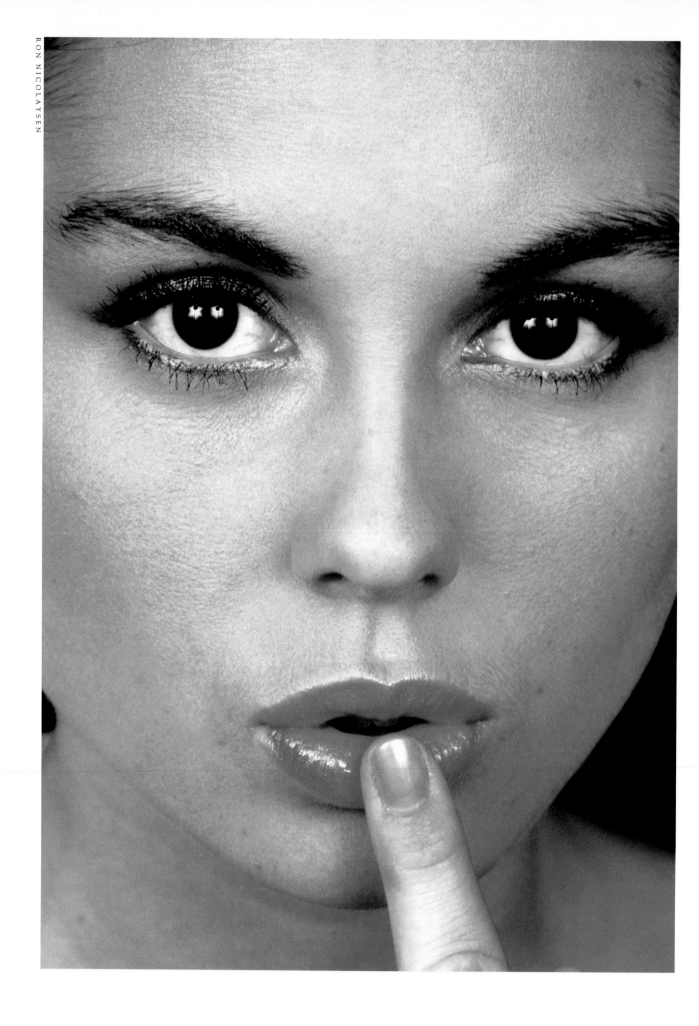

6

Luscious Lips That Last and Last

My Personal Philosophy About Lip Color

Lip color is meant for lips—not for front teeth, wineglasses, people's cheeks after a peck or a gentleman's shirt. Unfortunately, lipstick has a habit of forgetting its place and wandering off to those taboo spots. That's my gripe against it. Plus the fact that, unless you're very careful about how you apply it, you'll end up with much too much color—the old Bette Davis *Whatever Happened to Baby Jane?* mouth disaster!

Although I do think there's a place for lipstick—at night, well blotted and topped with shimmer; applied with a brush, when you want more intensity or as a touch-up during the day—I'm recommending another method for making your lips lightly vibrant.

Kathy Martin
The ultrakissable mouth

Pencil Me In

*Y*es, I'm a pencil man, all the way. Once you learn how to use lip pencils, you'll become a convert, too. How can you not? Lip pencil doesn't come off on things and it creates and retains a lasting shape. If you use the colors I recommend, you can create a mouth that is truly classic.

Cinnamon and Sienna: The Dynamic Duo

*M*y classic lip wardrobe for every woman, regardless of coloring (with the exception of olive and dark skin, which I'll cover separately) and for any hour of the day or night, consists of only two colors: cinnamon and sienna. Used correctly, which means properly applied and skillfully blended, this fabulous combo will enhance the natural tone of your lips while adding the slightest hint of vibrancy and finish.

There's nothing more attractive than moist, soft, healthy-looking lips, stained—not saturated—with color. Here's how you achieve it.

How to Use Lip Pencils

- Take up the cinnamon, which has a caramel tone, and apply it as you would lipstick on a brush, to shape the mouth and color it in.
- Once you've done that, go to the sienna pencil, which has a peachy cast containing some orange. It'll give your mouth color and warmth.
- With the sienna pencil, color the entire lip area, over the cinnamon, with a light stroke.

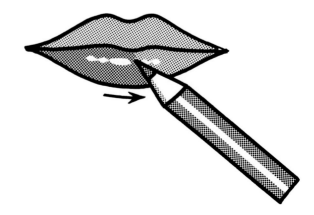

- Next, using a dry lipstick brush, blend the two colors until they have the uniformity of a single-color lipstick.
- Make sure you use dry pencils to get that marvelous classic matte finish and so the gleam from your lips doesn't blind anyone.
- If you want to add the slightest hint of moisture to the matte finish, use a lip balm or a sheer, opalescent lip gloss applied with a dry brush to make the bottom lip look sexily pouty, or "rolled."
- For daytime, make sure you restrict the gloss to the bottom lip; too much lip gloss all over looks messy and, well, a little cheap.
- For evening, as you've learned in the color charts, I like to use a little gold

ROBERT BROWNE

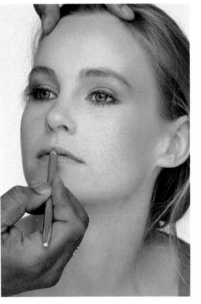

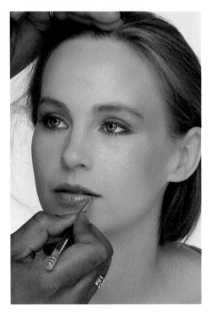

Here I'm giving Lisa Ryall lip—in the nicest possible way. First, with a sienna pencil to outline, color in and provide support for the darker pencil, which adds color. Then I'm adding the famous roll to the center of the bottom lip with gloss. Doesn't it look fabulous? Remember, by the way, that what applies to face contouring in terms of light and dark colors— one for shading, one for color—applies equally to the lips.

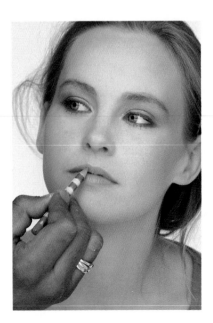

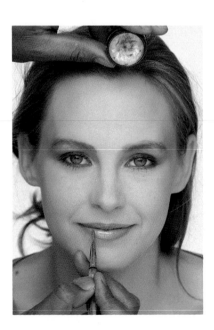

shimmer powder, mixed with gloss, to make the bottom lip seem "rolled." It's that "rolled" look which is responsible for those luscious moist mouths you see in magazines or movies.

Here's a great tip for dark lips: Use a dark brown eyebrow pencil to fill in any lighter parts of the lips, then add your color over it. Black women: Keep in mind that though you're able to use more emphatic colors, you must use them carefully—a too dark or too red color on the lips will be obvious, unless you're dressed up, since on you a lipstick-look always looks evening. The colors that are natural to you are true reds, burgundies, purples and maroons.

• For olive or dark skin, you'll be using a burgundy to mahogany pencil for shaping and a red-toned one over it.

Solutions to Special Problems

If Your Lips Are Thin

Rely on "overlining" to make your lips appear fuller, in which case your lip pencil becomes a superimportant tool. When you overline, go slightly outside your natural shape—without being obvious and looking like a clown—concentrating on the center section of the top lip and gradually tapering to the sides. Then fill in with the same color.

Be sure to "dot" on the line, rather than "drawing" a harder-edged shape.

The bottom lip will be slightly more exaggerated, mainly in the center. Remember, you're going for that full, sexy "roll."

If Your Lips Are Too Full

Think of Sophia Loren or Mick Jagger—there are worse problems to have than this, believe me! If you're bothered by your sensual lips, lip pencils are a step toward toning down because they avoid calling attention to imperfections that lipstick can't avoid. Lipstick states, lip

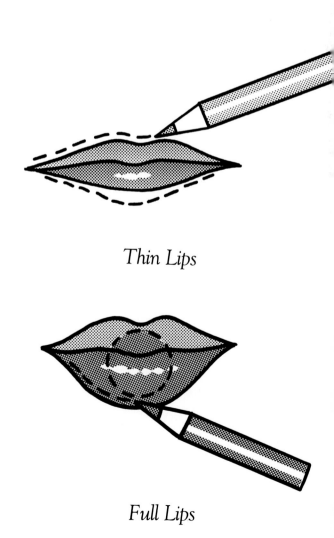

Thin Lips

Full Lips

pencil suggests and camouflages! To make your lips look less full, start with your lower lip and slightly line inside the natural perimeter, tapering off at the corners. Subtly shape your upper lip, making sure most of the color is concentrated at the center.

If Your Lips Are Wrinkled or Crinkly

Always use a moisturizer before applying color to help minimize wrinkling, and steer clear of lipstick—it's too heavy and will accentuate what you want to hide. After applying your pencil, use a cotton ball to add a touch of transparent powder to soak up any remaining moisturizer and to prevent color from bleeding. Really, you'll be amazed at how effective lip pencils can be for preventing bleeding, splitting, cracking or running.

If Your Lips Are Droopy or Turned Down

You'll be playing up the center of your mouth by keeping color in the middle of both the upper and lower lip. Never take the color all the way to the corners! If your mouth is too small or "droopy," you can "overline" lips slightly, using pencil at the outermost edges.

If Your Lips Are Puckered

Extend the lips away from the center toward the outer edges to create the illusion of pointy corners, but only from the bottom lip. You'll be creating length you never imagined you could achieve! How do you apply this? Just open your mouth and smile, and then create the corner that is barely there!

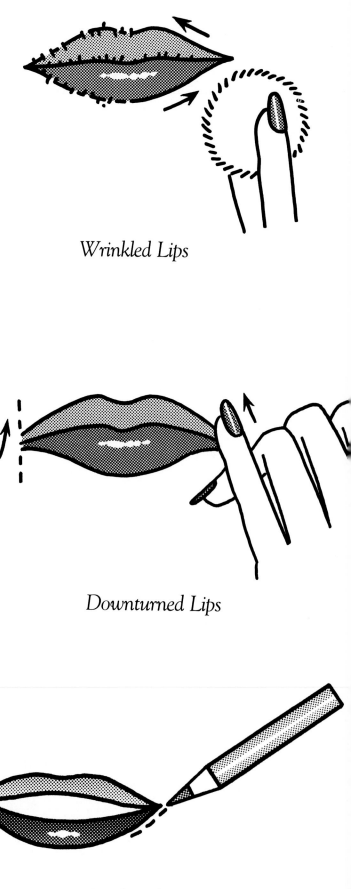

Wrinkled Lips

Downturned Lips

Puckered Lips

Nobody Doesn't Love Lip Pencils

*A*nd that includes you. Once you master the basics of working with this soft, "stainy," natural-looking lip glow, and choose from the charts the most flattering personal colors, you'll find yourself using lipstick only for afternoon touch-ups (make sure it is the same as your pencil).

Practical Magic

I know it's hard to believe, but that *is* your face. Honestly, that's what you really look like! You're not dreaming. You haven't been seeing visions. Well, yes you have, but they're visions of an oval face you can conjure up in a matter of minutes—sixteen to be exact —along with hypnotizing eyes and an irresistible mouth. And it's all in the next chapter!

ROBERT BROWNE

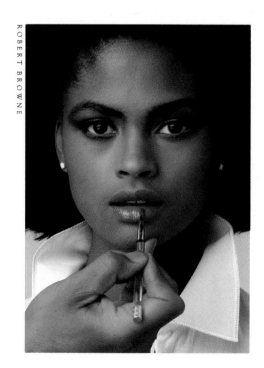

That roll to the bottom lip I keep talking about— where you put just a bit of gloss on the center of the bottom lip, here's how you do it. This time, I did it to Karen Alexander.

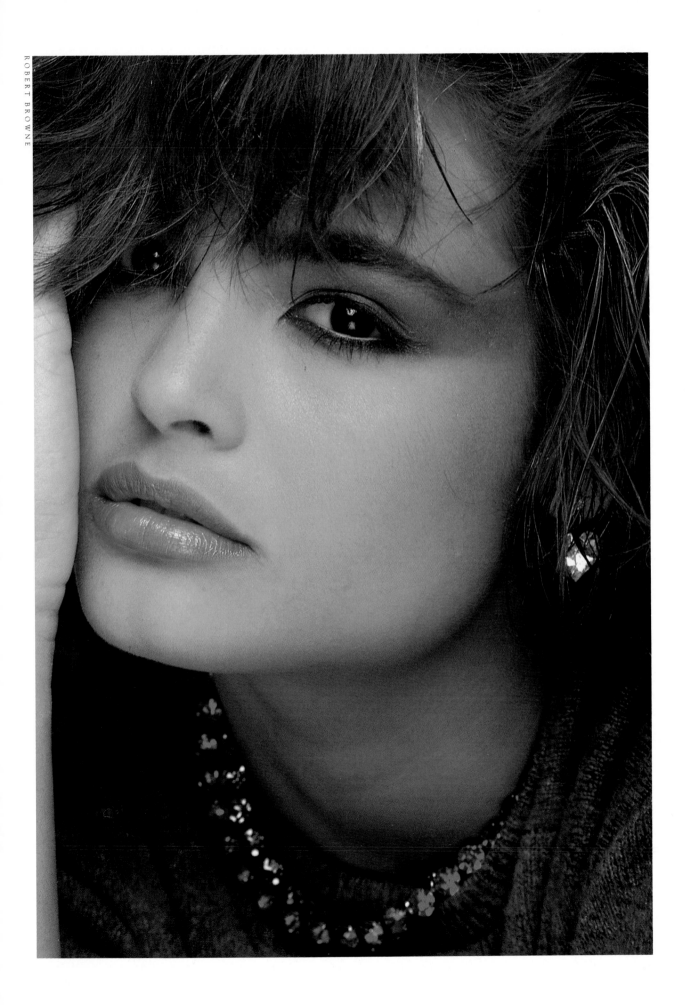

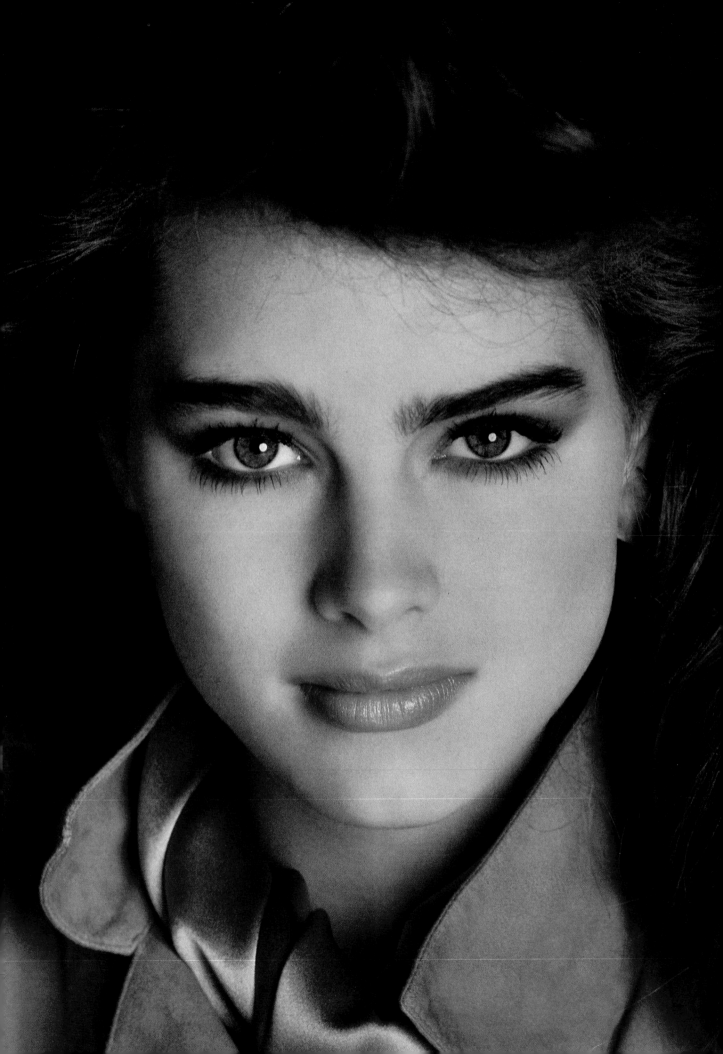

Part Three

The Only Makeup Guide You'll Ever Need

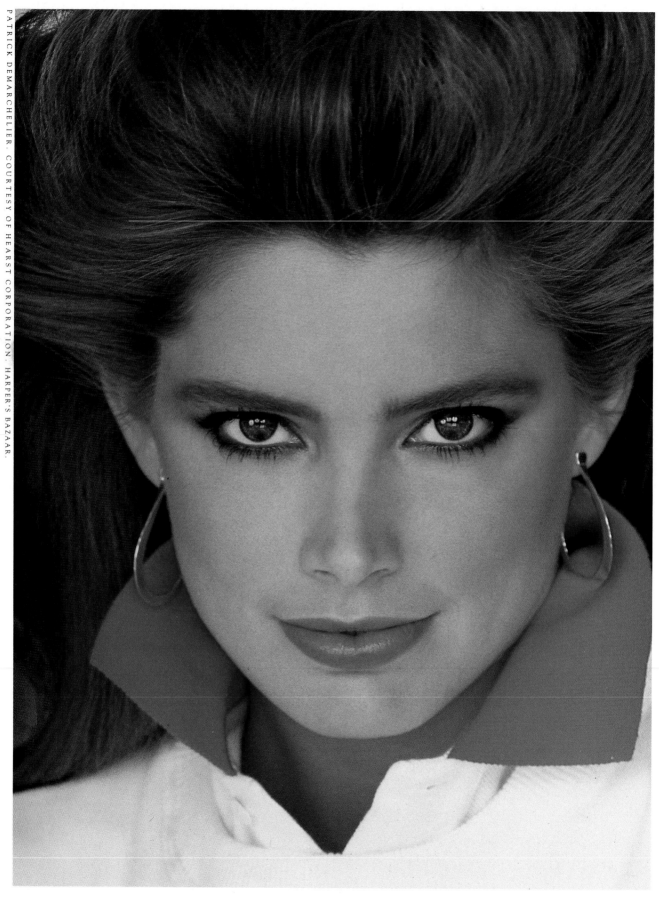

7

The Sixteen-Minute Makeup That Stays on from Morning to Night

Sixteen Minutes to Natural Glamour

The perfect eyes, mouth, cheeks, face—you can now create them all, feature by feature. But that's only the beginning. What you are going to master next is putting all the individual steps together into a routine that's going to become part of your life.

Sixteen little minutes is all it takes, but the benefits go on forever. And once you've practiced the basic routine, not only can you reduce the time it takes from sixteen to maybe eight minutes, you can also use variations that take even less time or more daring, depending

upon what aspect of your self-image you want to showcase to the world. Jogging, negotiating, at tea or in the wee small hours at a chic night spot, you'll look great while still maintaining your busy schedule and your classic essence.

You're simply too savvy—and too busy—to sit around all day and *paint* your face. You're going to learn how to *style* it, starting here, starting now.

Let's start with a recap of the basic materials you'll need. The things you'll have to have with you at all times are:

Kelly Emberg
Light and lovely beauty
that's practically instant

1. A light moisturizer (I prefer something with aloe);
2. A light transparent base (carry a little bit of it in a plastic vial that will fit in your purse or attaché case for patch ups and personal makeovers);
3. A tiny container of loose powder;
4. Your favorite rouges, one for contouring, one for color (when you're out, you can probably get along with your favorite color);
5. Mascara (let's stick to black or navy); one or two basic eye shadows or a set with complementary colors;
6. Two lip pencils (probably cinnamon and sienna) unless it's for evening, in which case, check the color chart for additional, more dramatic options—it's your decision;
7. Lip moisturizer;
8. Two fat little brushes—one for powder, the other for color;

And exclusively at home, be sure you keep:

1. Your battery of makeup brushes, from full-length duster to eyeliner and brow comb;
2. Lots of moisturizer, including both day and night creams;
3. Cleanser and astringent or freshener (if your skin is dry, stick to the freshener);
4. A range of, let's say, the three classic eye shadow colors and one or two options, all selected carefully from the color chart— either individual choices, or, if you can find one with the right colors for you, a set.

Now, let's go. The basic plan here uses makeup "neutrals," the colors that work the most universally. For your own individual makeup, be sure to consult the color chart (but you can certainly practice with the colors you have around the house).

Who's That Woman?

*I*t's the greatest feeling to be noticed, and remembered, from only a brief impression. And not because your perfume fills the room or your eye shadow vibrates, but because of your natural glamour. Always remember this, and repeat it to yourself if necessary; it's a truth that will enhance your self-image the way classic makeup enhances beauty. *The drama comes from you; everything else is an accessory.* You don't, and don't want to, look like a carbon copy of your favorite movie star or the newest cosmetic ad. You want to look like

In the before, Bitten looks great, but she doesn't look finished. All features are good, but they need to be subtly enhanced. Look at the after. It says it all.

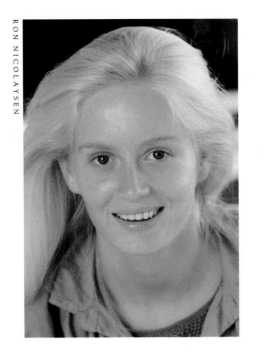

RON NICOLAYSEN

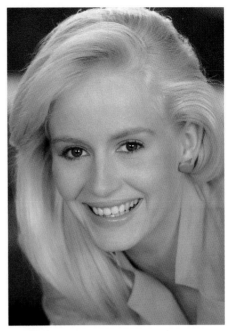

Lisa Ryall's a genuinely pretty woman, and by pretty I mean pretty, not perfect. She has a very high forehead. That's proof of intelligence, right? But it's also an opportunity to highlight an awful lot of facial flaws. Pay attention to how I've "smoothed" her skin, particularly in the area of the forehead. She has a naturally rosy cheek tone, so that was easy. All I had to do was take the basic pork chop shape and enhance it. Outside of that, all I've really done is . . . a lot, but it looks like I haven't done anything. She's got great equipment, but look how subtly I've accentuated her features to make her whole face glow!

ROBERT BROWNE

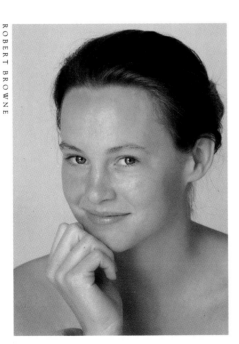

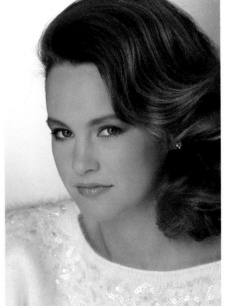

ART DIRECTOR: BARRY WEINBAUM. PATRICK DEMARCHELIER, COURTESY OF AVON PRODUCTS, INC.

Although it might take you a second to realize these are pictures of the same person, check again. I haven't tried to alter Melissa Gilbert's features; I've simply enhanced, smoothed and finished them. The pert nose is still the same in the after shot, as are the pert brow and neat little mouth but because color is subtly applied, the features stand out and the whole face glows.

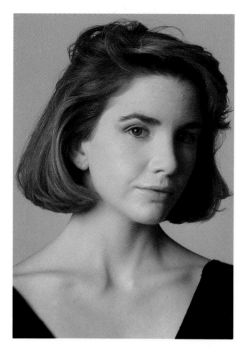
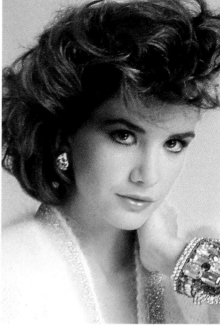

STAN WAN. COURTESY OF COSMOPOLITAN MAGAZINE, 8/84.

Beautiful daytime look on Carol Kurzin, from before to after. What I've done is pick up on the natural slant of the eyes, which is fabulous, and accentuate it. The contrast between the Asian sweep of the eyes and the American-ness of the rest of the face is really alluring.

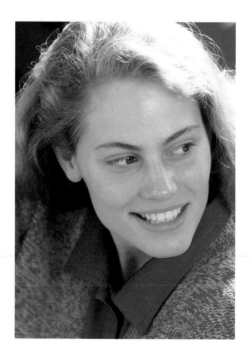
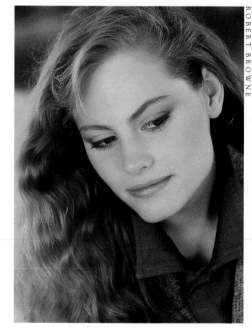

ROBERT BROWNE

yourself, facial idiosyncracies smoothed but never erased. You don't want to look perfect; you want to look perfectly lovely.

So here it is, my sixteen-minute program for making that lasting impression. In some cases, the step-by-step instructions will be more basic than what you've learned in the earlier chapters, but *basic* is the point of it. After we put the steps together into a system, I'll show you how to build on the basics to create a variety of looks with a greater range of complexity.

1. You've cleaned and moisturized, made a complexion inspection and taken care of anything you've found—blemishes, blotches, discoloration or wrinkles—with an undertoner.

2. With a damp sponge, dot on foundation, then sponge it in. Concentrate foundation on the areas that really need camouflage: the T zone—forehead, nose and chin.

3. If you still see valleys under your eyes, apply a cover cream *over* the foundation with a thin brush, start from the dark line by the bridge of the nose, then pat it lightly.

   Make sure moisturizer, foundation and cover cream are all perfectly blended!

4. Apply translucent powder with a cotton ball or puff and dust off any excess with a powder brush.

5. Now you're going to shape your eyes. Use a neutral shade, say caramel, on the entire lid area, from the base of the lashes up the lid, then apply a darker shadow from the middle of the lid, up along the crease, sweeping over and slanting up toward the brow and out toward the temple in an almond shape. If you'd like, apply a coordinated highlighter on the brow bone, but always make sure the shadows are evenly distributed and blended together, so they

look like one color on a more deep-set, larger, more dramatic eye.

6. Now frame your eye with a darker shadow liner, let's say teal or slate. Draw a line around your eyes with a moist thin brush, making the line heaviest at the outer triangle of the eye. Dry the brush with a tissue, run it through the dry shadow and repaint the line.

7. After shaping lashes with a curler, brush on navy or black mascara, wait ten seconds, brush eyelash comb through them, reapply mascara, wait another ten seconds and recomb. You'll know you're finished when there is no excess mascara balling on the lashes or bonding them.

8. Using your contour brush, apply toning rouge from the temple down the outer rim of the face to the cheekbone, stop the color directly below the iris of the eye. When finished, the rouge should resemble the shape of a pork chop.

9. Apply a peach rouge over a taupe, and blend the two with the color brush. Remember, the effect you're striving for is a lift to the entire face, so make sure you don't take the cheek color too close to your nose.

10. Outline and fill in lips with cinnamon and sienna lip pencils, applying the darker color first, then the lighter. Blend them; there should be no line of demarcation.

11. As you're looking for your keys, stop for a minute, reach in your purse and add a little shine to your lips with a balm or gloss. It'll give you a sexy "rolled" look.

    And that, as they say, is that. But from this humble beginning, I'm going to show you, through the magic of makeup, how to create three different versions of the classic you—all natural, all glamorous, all calculated to make you the sharpest woman on the block, no matter where you live.

Phoebe Cates

Before and After

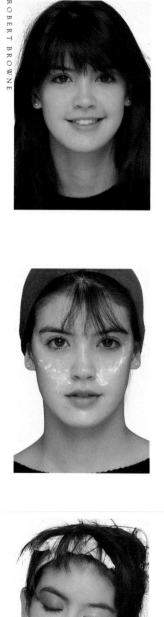

ROBERT BROWNE

*T*his adorable and exotic young actress/model—a real gamine, and the eighties equivalent of an Audrey Hepburn or Leslie Caron—is constantly working, not only as a model but also as a leading lady in the theater, on the screen (you remember her in *Gremlins*) and television (she played the title role in *Lace*). Phoebe's famous for her wholesome yet sultry looks, raven hair and porcelain skin, and for her classically lovely features—big doe eyes, angular nose, square jaw, oval face and that marvelous heart-shaped mouth. Now, let me tell you the whole story . . .

Here's Phoebe wearing no makeup at all. Actually, her very pale skin and very dark hair, being dramatic contrasts, tend to wash out her features. In addition, she has a petite, rather pointy face, even but not excessively strong eyes and nose, and a slight mouth. But we're going to change all that.

Phoebe's skin tends to be dry, even sensitive. So I dotted on *two* layers of moisturizer, making sure the first was absorbed, then the second. That extra layer of protection allows her makeup to glide on over the driest patches and gives her skin a dewy look.

To illustrate the enormous effect my classic makeup can have in correcting facial flaws, I did a half-and-half on Phoebe, making up only the right side of her face. Doesn't her eye look larger? Her face wider? Her jaw more sculptured? Her mouth more sensual?

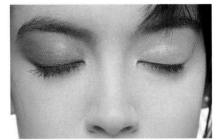

This half-and-half of Phoebe's eyes demonstrates a couple of my techniques. See how I've extended her browline and shadow out toward the temple, with the shadow curving up? Note how much wider her face looks and how much larger her eyelid seems. For her brow I've used a special trick exclusively for brunettes: I filled in the sparse areas in her brows with *auburn* pencil. That's an unconventional choice, since I almost always recommend going darker with brow pencil; but for a girl with hair as dark as Phoebe's, the use of the lighter pencil gives the entire face a lift.

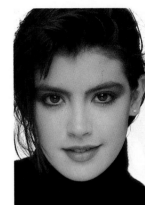

Here's a full shot of Phoebe's unusual daytime makeup, featuring her gorgeous eyes, her attention-getting hair, her pale skin and lovely features. Because of her alabaster complexion, I've selected gold-hued shadows that I'd normally use on a blonde and lined her eyes with olive liner (for evening, I'd suggest navy). Her color and shading rouges are both tones of sienna, which warm the whiteness of her skin. Notice that the rouge doesn't extend across her cheeks toward the nose. I've kept the color as a frame to widen her face and extended it high up toward the brow and subtly shaded it.

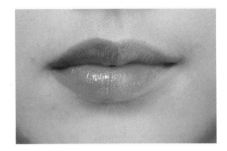

From this half-and-half, doesn't the right side of her mouth give the illusion of more generous, fuller lips? I got this effect by using just a bit of lip moisturizer in tandem with lightly applied lip pencil. Doesn't this "stainy" finish look luscious?

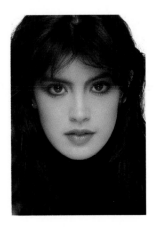

Here's Phoebe looking fabulous—the very dramatic way she's supposed to look when she's before a camera: healthy, vibrant, naturally stunning. And the tips she picked up from our working out her makeup—things like face shaping, lip coloring, and how to use eyebrows for emphasis and shadow as liner—she'll be able to incorporate into her off-camera, as well as her professional, life.

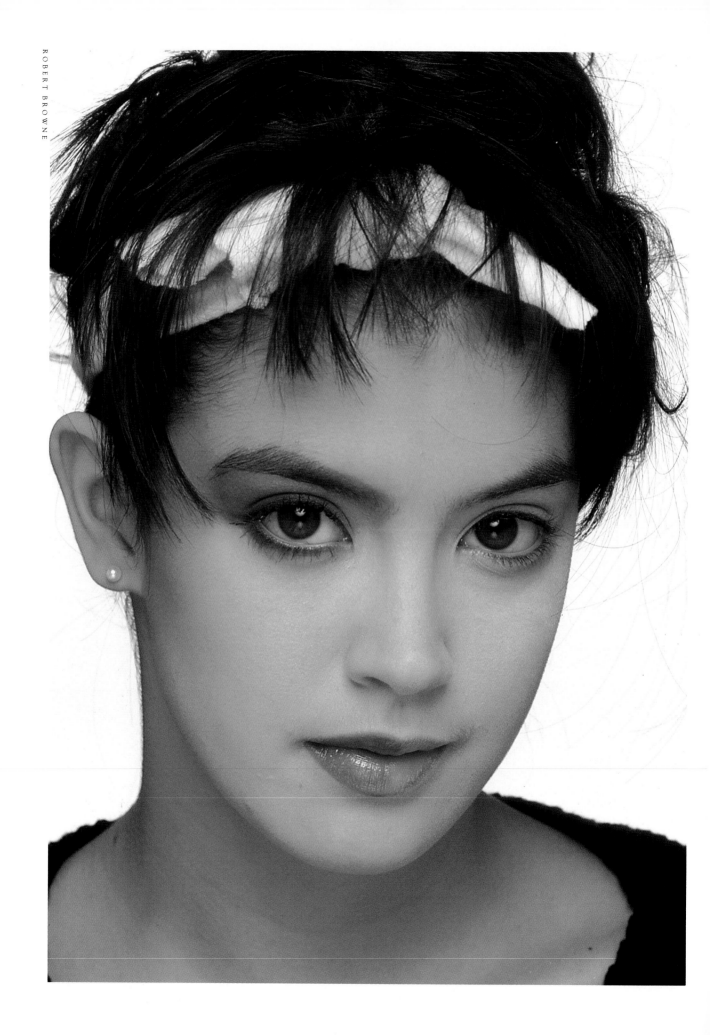

8

Touchups That Transform—

New Classic Beauty: From Weekend/ Sport Through Working Day to Fabulous Evening and Even Bedtime

Using the Twelve Basic Steps to Build Three Great Looks for Every Occasion

I appreciate how busy your life is, don't think I don't, and I know that sometimes you have to make the transition from marathon runner to business or household executive to glamour girl in almost no time at all. Gone are the days when a woman could spend hours at her dressing table, meditating over her eye shadow or shade of lipstick. Now you simply don't have time in your schedule for that. What you can do, though, is start with a simple, long-lasting everyday version of my sixteen-minute program, then learn how to transform yourself in seconds through the addition of a little more of this or that.

You'll always look classic, you'll always look fresh and upbeat, from morning to night, from Saturday evening to Sunday noon, and you'll do it so fast, people will think it's an illusion.

Phoebe Cates
Looking smashing on any
occasion

Working/Day Look

1. Since daytime is when we interact with people with specific goals in mind, eye contact is key; therefore, the working/daytime look is centered on the eyes. Here's where you'll apply several layers of mascara—being sure to let your lashes dry, then comb through them, before you apply the second layer. You must use shadow and liner now. If you don't, your eyes will look unfinished, and the mascara will actually cause them to jump out in an unattractive way.

2. Rouge is supposed to last all day, and to make sure it does, I'm going to tell you my secret for sealing color on your cheeks as long as you want.

  • After you've applied moisturizer and foundation, dust your face with translucent powder.

• Apply rouge, as you normally would, using the "pork chop" shape.
• Reapply translucent powder.
• Reapply rouge.
• If a glance in the mirror tells you you've overdone the color, you can always tone it down by adding a bit more powder. I guarantee your makeup will stay put until you decide to clean it off.
• A final reminder about blusher: What you're always trying for is an oval shape to the face.

  According to what you've learned in Part II, you'll be working to create an illusion: If your face is too wide, make your eyes look further apart; if it's too narrow, make them look closer. You'll also be trying to make your nose thinner and your lips fuller. I'm not promising that you'll end up looking like Liz

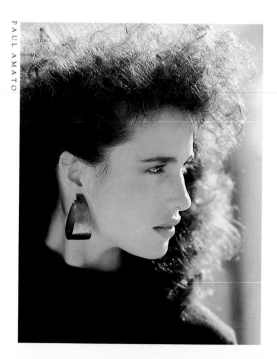

PAUL AMATO

If you're going to be seen in strong daylight, as Andie McDowell is seen here, make sure your makeup is well blended and that the color you use has just the right intensity. The best way is to make up in natural light. We can't all do that, but make sure you have the purest light source you can. That way, you'll have a good idea of how you're going to look when you greet the world.

Taylor, whose face is *the* perfect oval, but I can tell you that Isabella Rossellini, whose face appears to be oval, really has a "square" face—though with my makeup techniques you'd never know it.

3. In general, successful makeup depends on achieving the right depths and degree of color. You'll get it down to a science by experimenting with a little rouge, a little powder, a little more rouge, a little more powder, etc., until the color is strong enough yet soft enough to look finished and blended. And make sure it stops at the jawline!

4. For daytime, I'd recommend limiting lip pencil colors to the basic cinnamon and sienna, applied like lipstick. Start with the cinnamon to outline your lips, then use it to color and fill in. With a lip brush, "smear" the color so it "pales out." If you want to add more actual color, go over your lips with the sienna pencil, then lightly apply moisturizer to prevent a dry look.

5. I've said it before and I'll say it again: Dark skin and exotic looks call for more intense colors—rust, burgundy or copper lip pencils and blushers in burgundy, purple, magenta, red or cerise.

6. If you're running late or generally pressed for time and can't do a complete day makeup, here's what you do:

• First, apply moisturizer (mix in a bit of blush; it gives a lovely glow) and skip foundation, but spend a few extra minutes on your eyes, "framing" them with wet eye shadow and a little bit of mascara.

• The only additional items you'll need are moisturizer, a little rouge and lip color, but carry the rest of your makeup with you in case you want to enhance your look later in the day when you have more time.

• When the alarm didn't go off, and you've got to be in a meeting in half an hour, and you don't have time to do your eyes, here's a tip: Beautifully colored eyeglass frames with tinted lenses are a workable substitute for eye makeup. That way, you can do makeup in ninety seconds: moisturize, color your lips, slip on those specs and you're out the door!

Day and Night—a Major Difference

*T*he most serious cosmetic mistake most women make is to use the same makeup for evening and daytime. Stop it right now! Changing your hairstyle is not only enough, it's wrong. Your evening hairstyle shouldn't change substantially; what you do want to change is your makeup. Women don't seem to learn that too much makeup during the day ends up looking washed out at night; what they should do is use basically the same colors, but with more creative pizzazz for evening.

There's no doubt about it, wearing too little makeup is as big a mistake as wearing too much! And day and night makeup are as different as, well, day and night!

The Evening Look

*H*ere's where you're trying for a knockout effect, where you can try more dramatic eyes, cheeks and lips. But do you have to wash off your day makeup and start over?

1.　Make sure your evening makeup bag contains a couple of small shimmer eye shadows; a vial of shimmer powder; a slightly stronger lip color, say a soft red, depending on your coloring (check the color chart!), and a small container of a more intensely colored rouge. All this, by the way, fits into a small Baggie.

2.　To transform your face from day to night requires only these steps:

- Take your dry eye shadow and darken the outer corners of your lids, which, during the day, have a bisque-beige no-color hue, then smudge upward, giving the illusion of bigger eyes;

What if you don't have the chance or the time? I'm going to show you how to avoid a total reapplication and simply add to your day look:

- Reline your eyes using a wet shadow;
- Add a shimmery highlighter, perhaps a gold shade, under the brow;
- Apply a stronger cheek color, also chosen from the color chart;
- Do your lips with a more intense shade of pencil, then finish with a gold or metallic lip moisturizer;
- Give your hair a luxurious brushing; lightly dust your eyes, cheeks, arms, shoulders, décolletage with shimmer powder coordinated to your outfit, but within your skin tone, to give a pearly bronze glow, and you're ready to be ultraglamorous!

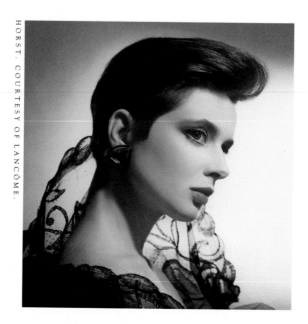

HORST. COURTESY OF LANCÔME.

Isabella Rossellini, conforming perfectly to my evening standards. Notice how the black lace of her dress casts a tawny tone to the exposed skin of her shoulders, which is echoed in the red in her hair and on her lips, the tawny on her cheeks and the golden alabaster of her skin. The eyes are in tones of black and glittering tawny-white. This is a perfect example of New Classic drama!

I always advise older women to avoid frosted shadows, even at night; they should concentrate on a really rich, warm brown for evening, or slate or charcoal gray on the outer corner of the eye and a warmer rouge and a brighter lip pencil! Exotic Black or Hispanic beauties can really go wild, with rouge and blusher in stunning, striking magenta, purple or even bright red!

Some Extra Supertips for Evening, Including What to Do When You Have Time to Start from Scratch

*O*nce you get the routine down to a science, you'll be able to add some of these hints and techniques to your evening look without also adding hours.

- Your makeup base doesn't have to be translucent; for evening occasions, it can "cover" because artificial light, as opposed to sunlight, calls for a more dramatic beauty statement. Put it over your day base or begin from scratch. Either way, keep in mind that at night, the most important element of your makeup is the eyes, with less color used on the face.
- Be daring and line your eyes with a gold or copper shadow, applied with a wet brush. Make sure the line you paint is close to the lashes, on both the upper

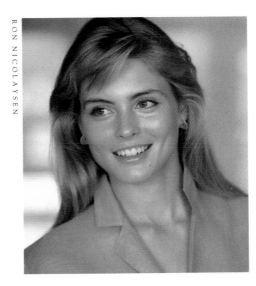

RON NICOLAYSEN

Kim's looking fresh and makeupless. But wait! She's actually wearing moisturizer, a very light blush and a lightly applied lip pencil with lots of gloss. But because this is the most casual of all looks, I've kept her eyes minimal so they won't spoil the clean, healthy, natural look of the whole face.

and lower lids. (In addition, if your skin is unwrinkled and can "take" it, you might want to think about a frosted blusher in copper, gold or bronze applied high on the cheekbones, over shoulders, cleavage, collarbones.)

- If you've got very dark eyebrows, for evening use a light eye shadow in the copper family—anything with a little red in it—and brush over the brows to control and soften them. If your brows are lighter, feather them in with pencil.
- For evening, contour takes on a whole different ambition for shaping the face. You don't want a rouged look because it's just too much, so play down cheek color and play up eyes and lips.
- Contouring isn't meant to be dark; it's meant to give the impression of natural shadow. For evening, what you want from contouring is *lift*, and to do that you'll keep color as far away from nose and cheeks as you can, applying it, instead, at the top of the cheekbones toward the temples.

- If you've got a thin mouth, add a little bit of gold gloss, but only to the lower lip. It makes the mouth look fuller and very, very lush.
- Older women especially must be sure not to duplicate daytime makeup for the evening. You should always make sure you have three distinct looks, which requires, for example, three different rouges: soft for weekends, neutral for daytime, stronger for evening. Check the color charts; they'll steer you in the right direction.

Weekend/Sport Face

*E*ven when you're dashing over to the supermarket, headed for an aerobics class at your health club or meeting a friend at the courts for an early morning tennis game, you can never tell who you're going to run into.

Just because the circumstances are informal, doesn't mean you shouldn't look your best. However, in this case, looking your best means looking your most natural.

Here's how:

1. Moisturizer's a must whether you're exercising at home or running a marathon. When you're exerting yourself physically, the skin tends to become taut; a moisturizer, especially one with aloe, will really help counteract that effect. As always, make sure your moisturizer is completely absorbed before leaving the house. If you do, you'll avoid a greasy-feeling face and allow your pores to sweat freely.

2. The essence of this look is understatement, and the object of the makeup is a monochromatic, natural face with just a bit of glow. You'll achieve this by applying blusher (if you're going to be exerting yourself, use cream, rather than powder rouge; it won't streak from perspiration) over your cheekbones, on your eyelids instead of shadow and on your forehead; then it's powder, lightly dusted over your

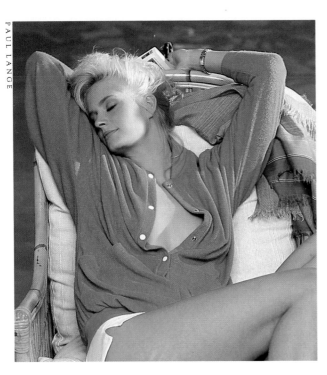

PAUL LANGE

Weekend/Sport

If you want to stay in the swim makeupwise, apply waterproof mascara very, very lightly before plunging into the pool or the ocean. In terms of base, I'd steer toward a colored moisturizer, which you can use as a "color wash" over your entire face, or to highlight cheeks and temples, and also very lightly, add lip pencil. This will wash off slightly, but that will only make you look more natural. Frankly, if you're deep-sea diving or doing laps, don't count on emerging with much left on your face. But for sitting around a pool, it's great!

skin so you look as if you're very faintly blushing.

If you're using cream or gel rouge or bronzing, try this: Mix a small amount of color into your moisturizer, which you then apply as usual, to give your skin an all-over glow. Blondes should stick to peach tones of blusher, brunettes to rosier colors, and exotic types to richer colors, such as burgundy, mahogany or garnet.

3. The only other makeup you need for your informal face, then, is a little mascara, some undereye cream or a light foundation, applied only where you really need it, and lip moisturizer, either with or without color.

And that's about all there is to it, except for special cases.

Après-Exercise Touchups

1. After you've showered, be sure to remoisturize, mix some cream blush in with it, but this time take a little more care about shaping your face, which means subtly applying additional blush in that pork chop shape—never in a straight line, and never moving toward the nose—so your face looks natural but finished. No red circles on each cheek, please!

2. Put a little blusher on your lid, then apply your mascara and as much lip color as you want; now you're ready to go.

The Bedtime Look

*W*ould you believe makeup you can sleep in? Let's face it, there are times when you want to wake up looking natural, with just the slightest, sexiest hint of enhancement. Here are some tips for a very light-handed, natural look that's *un*painted, *un*done, with just a glimmer of color—and he'll never know it's makeup!

- Whatever you do, don't use anything on your face that will smear on your pillow. That's messy—and a dead giveaway.
- To brighten skin tone, apply color to the cheeks by mixing rouge with moisturizer and just grazing it on and over the cheeks, blending it until it's just barely visible. Make sure it dries!
- Don't use powder at all; it creates too finished a look and it can come off on pillows.
- Apply just a touch of lip pencil, then rub most of it off to add the barest impression of natural stain.

That's it. Remember, you're not trying to look made-up, so don't use mascara; you're trying to look fresh, healthy and natural!

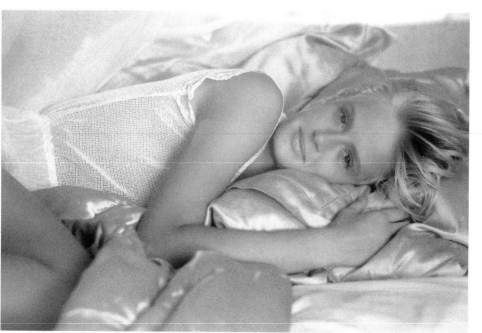

PAUL LANGE

Bedtime's an occasion, so why not try a makeup designed especially for times when you've got to look natural but when you also want to look your best—very close up. You want to impart a blush, no more than that. Here I've lightly colored Bitten's cheeks and lips with a hint of color and left the eyes perfectly natural.

My Reader, the Makeup Artist

*D*id I lie? Is this system not easy? And classic? And flattering? Life is simply too short to waste time, even on yourself, and now you don't have to. With New Classic Beauty, you can eliminate a long and often frustrating part of your day, one that leaves you still unsure if you've created the right face for the occasion. And be honest with me? Don't you look terrific? But so subtly it's hard to spot why.

When people ask, say you're in love, it never hurts!

In the next couple of chapters I deal with two groups that are different from the rest of you in the makeup area. Your color rules don't apply to them: women over forty and exotic types, such as Black, Hispanic, Asian and olive-skinned women.

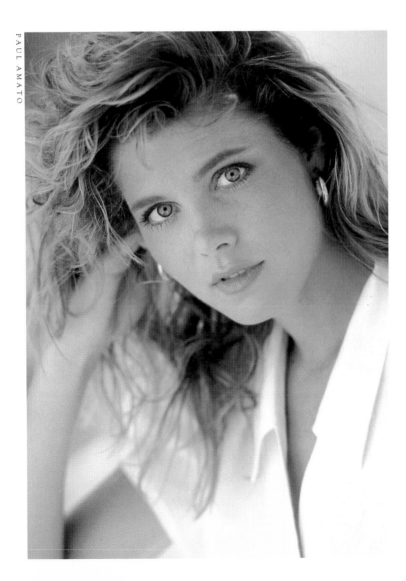

PAUL AMATO

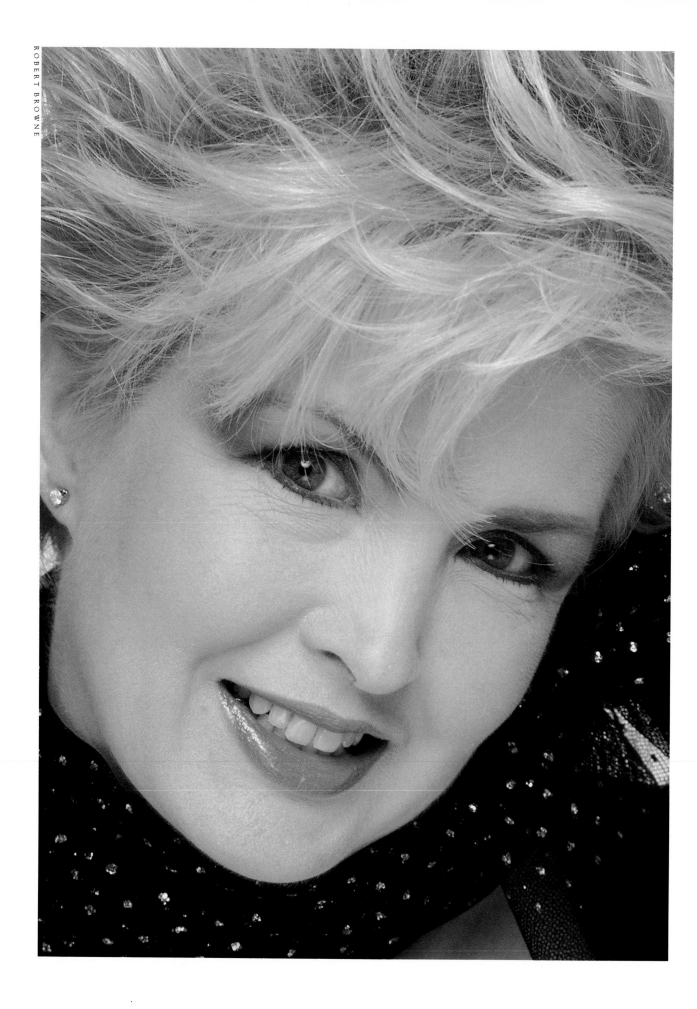

9

Glamour After Forty

A Second Chance at Colors!

These days, age really is becoming a state of mind, so don't talk to me about how depressing it is to get older. That is simply not allowed. Especially when being over forty is absolutely no excuse for letting yourself get out of shape or look drab. Look at Elizabeth Taylor, Jane Fonda, Margaret Thatcher, Barbara Walters! You know why so many more women are looking better longer? Remember, you heard it here! It's because women have more power, more freedom to develop their essence, their self-image—whatever you want to call it. Their presence is responsible for their success, and they know that presence comes from inside. As you age, you adjust your style but you never change it. It would be like having your face surgically reconstructed as that of another person rather than a lift of your own features!

Aside from that, getting older really can be liberating. You know your established place in the world, you can face the fact that you've accomplished something in your life, and now you can enjoy it.

Makeup is part of that enjoyment because, now that your face and hair require a softer look, you get a whole new set of colors and rules to play with. After years of being a cute brunette, you're about to become an elegant silver-haired woman of a certain age—the absolute *epitome* of chic! I want to recapture the glow your face expressed at twenty-five, but not your twenty-five-year-old makeup. I want to enhance your spirit, your personality, those things that don't change, and with such subtlety, such finesse, you'll dazzle yourself!

As women get older, they need to update their makeup along with their wardrobe, learning to apply cosmetics proficiently. It's never

Barbara Alexis
Classic means forever

too late to learn—or to improve—so, despite your years, you've got to practice applying cosmetics regularly, and to choose the right colors to avoid emphasizing the lines and puffiness that can occur around the eyes.

Makeup, regardless of your age, can enhance your style and truly change your looks. Here are some tips I've collected on how to showcase your natural glamour whether you're forty, fifty or more.

Skin Care After Forty

*A*s you know, to prevent the dryness that comes with age, you should use moisturizer all the time and all over your face, giving special attention to the eyes, neck and throat with "target" creams directed to the particular area. In addition:

- Remember that getting enough sleep discourages bags and dark circles under the eyes.
- Avoid puffiness by making sure your bedroom is not overheated, use a humidifier during the winter and sleep with your head slightly elevated so fluids "move" down and away from the face.
- Stay away from salty foods, which retain water in the body; cigarettes and alcohol, which dry out the skin and add to wrinkling. Take the sun only with maximum protection.
- A good remedy for puffiness: wet teabags applied to the eyes!
- When applying treatments or cosmetics, never "tug" at your skin; let them slide on to maintain a minimal loss of elasticity as long as possible.

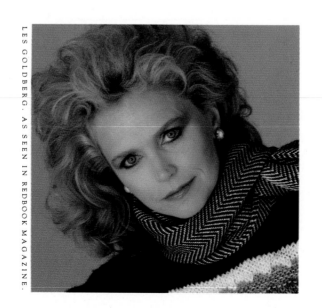

LES GOLDBERG. AS SEEN IN REDBOOK MAGAZINE.

The great thing about eyes: They never age, especially when they're as electric blue as Lee Remick's. They're the most galvanizing feature in her lovely face, so I played them up by lining them dark to bump up the whites which, in turn, makes the blue bluer.

Hints Toward a Flawless Finish

- The first thing to remember if you're over forty is to make sure your skin is sufficiently moisturized to "take" color, whether it's a cream or powder. Since skin dries as you age, preparing your face is even more important than ever.
- When applying foundation, which is matched to the natural skin color of your neck, don't use it all over your face. Apply it in spots—say, your forehead, cheeks, above your upper lip and on your chin—and blend it very, very well to avoid a masklike look.
- Make sure you use little or no foundation on areas where your skin is most wrinkled, and never around the eyes if you're wrinkled there (makeup tends to settle in lines and wrinkles, making them more pronounced).
- Make sure you apply foundation (cream for dry skin, water-based if your skin is oily) with a damp silk sponge to "sheer out" base without tugging. For added sheerness, mix your foundation with moisturizer, then apply and blend in; for a healthy, natural glow, add a bit of bronzing gel to the base and moisturizer.
- To minimize undereye circles and lines, use a lighter foundation or undereye cream, applied by mixing it first with moisturizer, for better "slide" over delicate eye skin, then pat on.
- To minimize the lines extending from your nose to your mouth, sparingly apply a lighter foundation, an undereye cream or a white pencil, which goes *under* your regular foundation.
- Remember that powder looks best when applied sparingly, so be sure to dab it on with a puff then brush off any excess, thus ensuring the sheerest possible coverage. Don't use powder in problem areas; it'll only cake in lines and make your skin look drier. Especially for older skin, the purpose of translucent powder is to keep the shine away from your face; the desirable shine should come from the hair.
- Don't use anything glittery or iridescent around the eyes or on the lips. Keep in mind that matte finishes minimize, while sheen reflects and magnifies.
- If your eyes are puffy, use the darker eye shadow colors recommended in the charts to provide the illusion of shadow and depth.
- If your lips "bleed" because of fine lining, use a little powder over them, then outline the lips with a freshly sharpened pencil. That way, when you apply color, you'll be able to fill in a more precise shape.
- A fuller, more natural brow is an instant "youthener," so be sure to brush brows upward, enhancing their maximum shape, then fill in with a "no-color" toned pencil, which you'll feather, rather than stroke on.

Why Hair Is Even More Crucial as You Get Older

*C*ut, care, color—three little words that spell glamour whether you're turning forty or have passed the sixty mark. Before I give you my own tips, though, a few words of advice: Don't be penny-wise and pound-foolish, which is to say, don't choose a salon because it's close or because you've been going there for years. Also, don't go to a friend's hairdresser just because you like the style of her cut; chances are, if the stylist gave you the same cut, it wouldn't be right. Bring a picture if you want, even book yourself for a consultation and meet with the artist, then go home and think about it. If you like what the person had to say, make an appointment; it's worth the extra pennies, believe me. Now, hints:

• As a rule, shorter hair works better on women over forty. If your hair is fine, a blunt, straight cut will flatter you; if your hair is thick and wavy, I'd recommend something layered. Unless you have it styled every day, a mane can be aging to an older woman because it "drags down" your features. Wearing your hair up is often too severe, but so is overly short hair. The secret of hair as a fashion accessory for the woman over forty is not to be extreme—too far off the face is overly done, too far forward is overpowering.

• Hair, like skin, dries out—and thins—as we age, and as hair loses color, the texture changes, becoming coarser and more flyaway. To counteract the unmanageability that hair may display as you move past forty, make sure you get a good cut in a style you can manage yourself, a look you and the stylist have discussed and agreed on before scissors touch your locks. And if you wash your hair every day, be sure to dilute your shampoo, regardless of what it says on the directions!

• To add volume and fullness, I recommend applying setting lotion or gel while your hair is still wet, then comb it through. When you begin to blow-dry, bend at the waist so your hair falls forward, and brush it toward your face. When you've dried your hair enough so that it's still damp but not wet, comb it into place and let it dry naturally.

• I believe in coloring hair, no doubt about it, especially now, when coloring techniques are so much more varied and so much less damaging. The new conditioner-colorings actually wash in richness and sheen, while new methods of blonding brighten and highlight hair naturally. Never forget, the aim of hair color is not to change your natural color, but to enhance it.

• If you're concerned about going gray, you might want to try reverse streaking, highlighting or a color rinse, which is temporary, but I don't advise doing it yourself.

Please, please, place yourself in the hands of a qualified expert. He or she can give you what you want better than you can, believe me!

A Stunning New You!

*A*fter years of using the same old colors, you're getting permission to go on to a whole new look. That is supposed to give you an incentive not to miss that aerobics class, to urge you to stop smoking or doing anything else that works against staying young and fresh! These days you can look great in your eighties, so don't you want to be around, still looking fabulous? Remember, a woman who was "cute" at thirteen isn't often "cute" at fifty, but a well-groomed, elegantly made-up, self-confident woman of any age will be handsome as long as she lives.

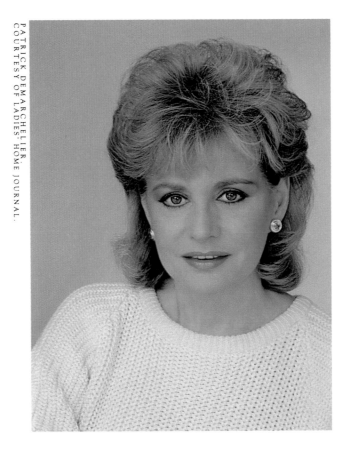

PATRICK DEMARCHELIER; COURTESY OF LADIES' HOME JOURNAL.

For Barbara Walters's eyes I went light, using neutral tones and minimal mascara. Her shadow is matte, because women over forty should never wear shimmer shadow: It calls attention to lines and wrinkles. The one exception to that rule is highlighter under the brow. Her blush is actually used more for contour than actual color, and her lips, while they do have color, don't stand out.

Barbara Alexis

The makeup I did on Kim Alexis's mom, Barbara, is a textbook example of makeup for women over forty. In the first shot, I've mixed classic blue undertoner with moisturizer to smooth her skin. Next, I'm applying undereye cream to where she has the most lining—under the eyes and from the nose to the mouth. After foundation, I've powdered her, mandatory for women over forty, because it prevents that oily shine that accentuates wrinkles and lines.

I've lifted her brows to the maximum because that raises the entire face and used subtly applied bronzy tones for the shadow, which is matte (remember, she's a blonde, so despite the fact that she's over forty, she'll still stay in the blonde, peachy, golden range colorwise). The olive shadow used as liner will actually be lightly applied because we don't want to call attention to the undereye wrinkles. Since mascara can be glaring on older women, I've given Barbara's eyes drama mainly by using shadow applied as liner with a wet brush. She doesn't have much lip wrinkling, but her mouth, while small, is a little tight. Through using some color, but not a lot, I've given her mouth size, moistness and a more subtle definition. Here's Barbara's finished evening makeup—dramatic, colorful, but not overstated in the least. Her skin looks glowing and whatever lining or creasing she has on her face really isn't noticeable. Of course, it never hurts to be beautiful to begin with.

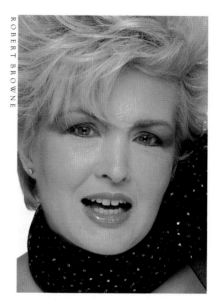
ROBERT BROWNE

ROBERT BROWNE

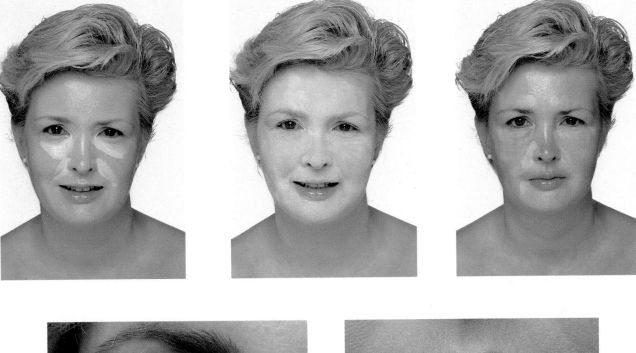

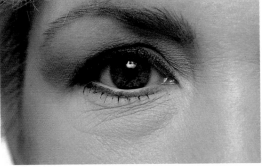

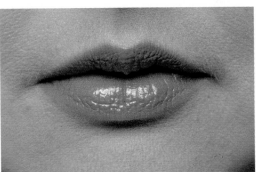

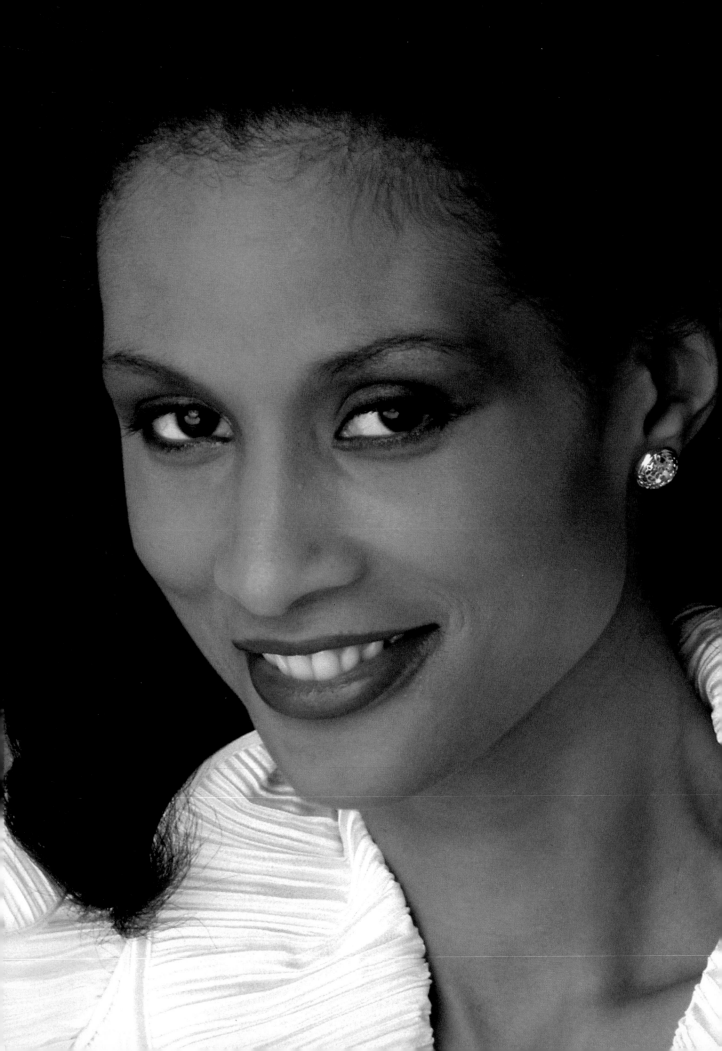

10

If You're an Exotic Type . . .

For Women Who Are Hispanic, Black, Asian or Deep Olive-Skinned

Exotic, in the makeup world, means any skin color range that requires special rules and combinations—and offers a chance to enhance your natural glamour that your more pale-toned sisters will never have! You alone can project your strong, self-confident image through bright color—red lipstick, burgundy blusher and lip colors to die from! If you're Black, Hispanic, Asian or have the deep-olive Mediterranean look of Isabella Rossellini, these tips are for you!

Beverly Johnson
The utter glamour of
real color

Foundation and Undercreams for Exotics

• If you have more yellow in your skin tone than you'd like, counteract it with green veil undertoner on a cover-up brush before applying moisturizer and your foundation with a sponge. It'll make the sallowness disappear like magic!

• If you have more gray in your skin tone than you want, use the classic blue undertoner; it'll brighten your skin perfectly.

• Check the color chart for the foundation pairings that seem right for you. Foundation pairings for lighter-skinned women, including many Hispanics and Asians, are medium beige to tawny beige. (For sallow skin, use over an undertoner. The tawny color, sometimes called "luggage," is a golden-yellow rust, and what you'll get is a beautiful golden tone but no sallowness.)

If your skin is darker olive to medium brown, you'll fall into the deep olive to toasted honey range. If your skin is very dark, you'll use desert tan, alone or with chocolate.

• All the other rules of applying foundation given in the earlier chapters apply to you: Blend the two base colors to achieve a perfect tone that matches the skin on your neck.

• Remember, always use moisturizer, even if your skin is oily.

• Your undereye cream will almost always be in the medium to dark range.

• If your skin tone has a silvery, ebony cast, try classic blue undertoner, and if it is tawny, with a lot of yellow, try green veil.

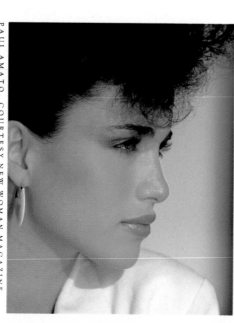

This utterly fabulous-looking olive-skinned beauty has smooth and beautiful skin, but it tends to have a more intense yellow cast than she'd like. What I did was apply green undertoner all over her face before blending foundations and applying them. In doing that, I changed "sallow" to "tawny." Doesn't her skin radiate a healthy, burnished glow? I kept the lip and cheek color in tones with a lot of tawny orangeness to complement the ravishing color of her skin.

Eyes for Exotics

- You alone get permission to use black liner! Since your skin is dark, you can, in almost every case, use intense colors to enhance your features. But you might want to try liners like deep olive or mahogany with coppery day tones.
- Think of the shadows you can use, even for day—royal blue, jade, garnet in addition to the basics—without looking overly made-up!
- Since your skin is darker, the whites of your eyes give a lot of natural intensity.

Play it up for evening by rimming the inside of your eyes with white eye pencil. It makes the evening eye stand out!
- For evening, keep in mind that your shadow is keyed to your hair, skin and eye color, while shimmer powder is coordinated with your outfit.
- If you're wearing a bare dress, dust shimmer powder over your arms, neck and shoulders. A little glow will bring out the beautiful lights in your skin tone!

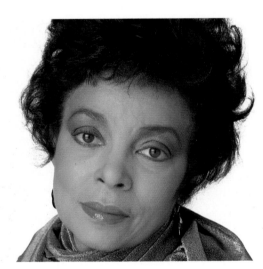 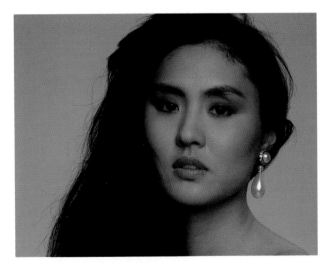

ROBERT BROWNE

Great actresses have great faces, and in their case, aging does add character. With the magnificent Ruby Dee, I didn't try to camouflage the character; I've simply smoothed it.

Your looks are naturally ultrastriking because of the intense contrast of your skin and hair. The whole world envies you your almond eyes, so accentuate their shape and lengthen them in dark liner (*you* can take it) and by perfectly blend-

ing shadows outward. If you have a complexion problem, it's sallowness, but by using green undertoner and properly blended bases, you can turn skin softly tawny or even a warm ivory, depending upon your natural tone. Since your

face has more organic color than many occidental brunettes, you can take stronger tint on the cheeks and lips. Remember your naturally dramatic coloring is your outstanding "accessory." Play to it!

Cheeks for Exotics

- Remember, blush is color. Contour is the way it's applied to the face—always in the shape of a pork chop, up and around the temples and right up to the hairline!
- Your contouring will be done in either dark bronze or mahogany—whatever's a tad darker than your skin.
- The only difference between

conventional coloring and coloring for exotics is intensity; the rule pretty much stays the same, but the colors shift to a higher gear. For your color blush, you might think of trying burgundy, purple or magenta, but watch a cherry red, it sometimes has a tendency to turn pink on dark skin.

Lips for Exotics

- On Blacks, lipstick almost always gives an "evening" look, which is another reason to use lip pencils. You can use essentially the same tone as your favorite lipstick, but it will last longer and look much more "stainy," much newer (fresher) looking.
- If your skin is light brown, olive or sallow, I'd stay away from intense colors and stick to a color in the copper or rose

family. It'll be soft, after being blended with gloss, and very fresh.
- If your lips have light and dark patches, apply a medium to dark contour cream under your gloss for ideal evenness.
- Once the sun goes down, you can go mad with lips! Just be sure it doesn't detract from your outfit, which, as we know, all evening makeup is designed to highlight.

Warning!

*R*émember this if you're an exotic: Because your skin has more color than most, it can take more color. That's great, but there's a catch! You're using brighter colors, but you have to learn to apply them with the same subtlety and elegance that everyone else does. Don't go overboard! As long as you don't, you'll be sailing along looking glamorous.

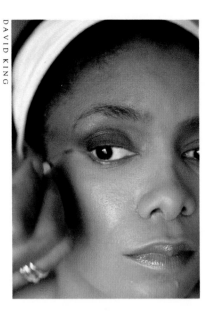

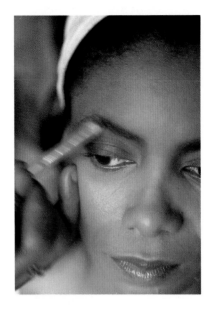

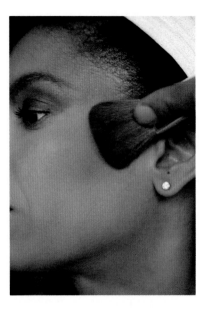

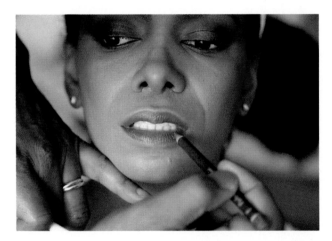

Here's one of my favorite examples of makeup for women with dark skin. After applying foundation that brings out the tawny golden quality of Darnella Thomas's skin, I've used a strong slate on her eyes, both as shadow and liner. Her blush is one of those wonderful colors only exotic types can wear—a real burgundy, but applied subtly, both for shaping and coloring.

I'm feathering in her brows where they're thinnest with a lighter color, to bring a lift to the eye and in fact the entire face, and I'm letting the lips make the kind of statement that only dark skins can make. Even so, this is daytime, striking without being assaulting.

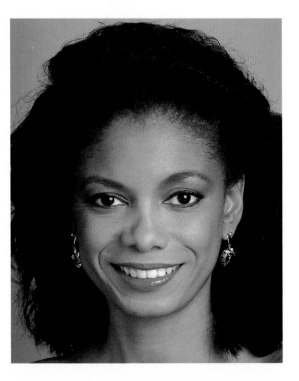

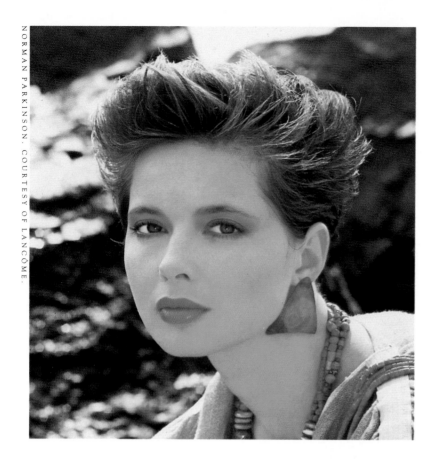

NORMAN PARKINSON. COURTESY OF LANCÔME.

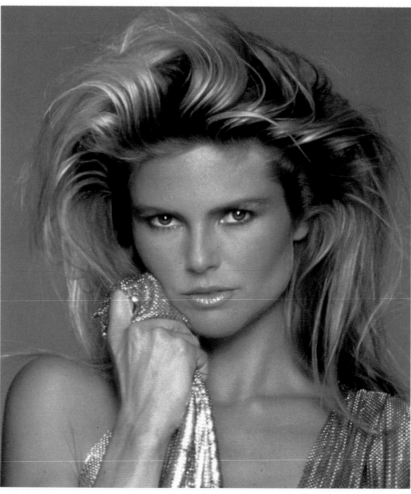

PATRICK DEMARCHELIER

Conclusion: You Were Never Lovelier!

So now you're about to graduate from the New Classic Beauty course. You've done terrifically well in the lessons and are ready to announce to the world that you're looking glamorous and natural. And it's taken you practically no time at all.

What you're going to find with New Classic Beauty is that not only will it make you look simply marvelous, it's also consummately economical—and not just with your time, but with your money, too. That's part of the classic standard; you don't have to buy a lot but what you buy has to be of excellent quality and not go out of style.

Never forget that you're a classic, too, with an essence that only you possess, and it doesn't change with the years. The aim of my makeup is to bring out that essence, whether you're fifteen or seventy, to downplay imperfections and enhance the glow that comes from inside you . . . always. You have natural glamour, and I've shown you how to highlight it. So go out there and knock 'em dead!

Here's Isabella Rossellini opposite Christie Brinkley. You can appreciate why she's an exotic. Next to really pale, she broadcasts her olive tones. In this photo, one of my favorites, the photographer is picking up on the olive skin by toning it down, by using an undertoner that takes out the bad yellow and makes her skin color coordinate the colors he's trying to sell.

Christie is a study in gold, which, let me remind you, is what I told you blondes should wear. The body in the bathing suit doesn't hurt, either.

Here, gold and olive serve the same functions, depending on your skin tone. Christie's gold is Isabella's olive.

In order to help you select the perfect makeup for you, we are repeating the color
charts on perforated paper. Just tear out the
sheet for your coloring and carry it with you for
easy reference while you are shopping.

Foundation from A to Z

Undertones

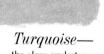

Green Tone—
the fairest of skins

Turquoise—
the class undertoner
for all skin tones

Highlights
undereye cover

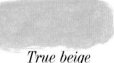

Light medium

Medium to dark

Foundation

Pure ivory

True beige

Light beige

Light medium beige

Medium beige

*Tawny tan
(yellow skin type)*

Deep olive

Toasted honey

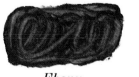

Desert tan

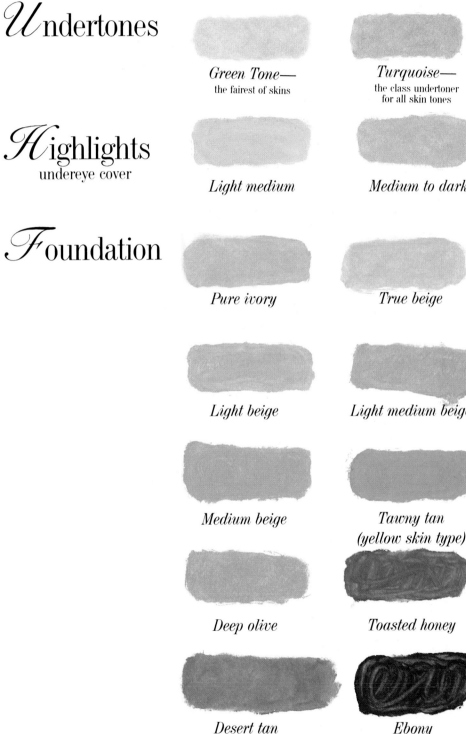

Ebony

Chocolate

Shimmer Powders

Opalescent

Silver

Gold

Fuchsia

Bronze

Slate

Dark bronze

Brunettes

Eyes

Rust   *Bronze*   *Slate*

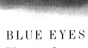

BLUE EYES
Classic brown

GREEN EYES
Soft gray

HAZEL EYES
Mushroom

BROWN EYES
Classic navy

DARK BROWN EYES
Olive

Cheeks # Lips

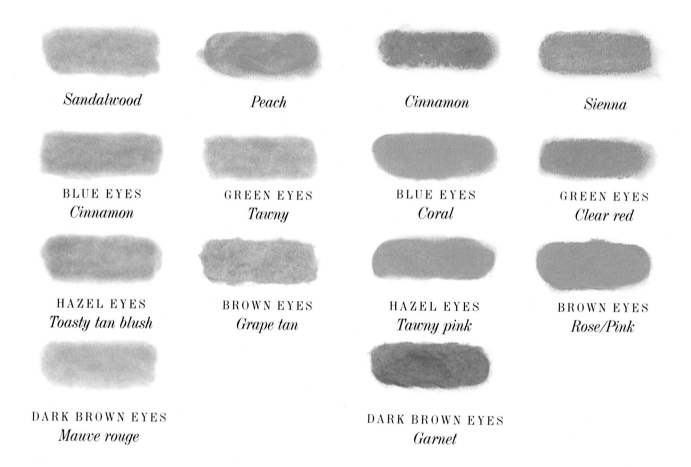

Sandalwood

Peach

Cinnamon

Sienna

BLUE EYES
Cinnamon

GREEN EYES
Tawny

BLUE EYES
Coral

GREEN EYES
Clear red

HAZEL EYES
Toasty tan blush

BROWN EYES
Grape tan

HAZEL EYES
Tawny pink

BROWN EYES
Rose/Pink

DARK BROWN EYES
Mauve rouge

DARK BROWN EYES
Garnet

Blondes

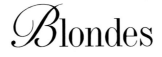

Eyes

Light gold

Dark gold

Terra-cotta

BLUE EYES
Slate

GREEN EYES
Classic peacock

HAZEL EYES
Mustard brown

BROWN EYES
Classic burgundy

DARK BROWN EYES
French blue

Cheeks

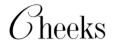

Soft bronze

BLUE EYES
Cinnamon

HAZEL EYES
Sandalwood

DARK BROWN EYES
Sienna

Classic peach

GREEN EYES
Creamy cocoa

BROWN EYES
Pale mauve

Lips

Cinnamon

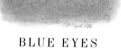

BLUE EYES
Natural beige pink

HAZEL EYES
Pale peach

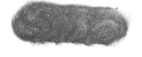

DARK BROWN EYES
Golden cider

Sienna

GREEN EYES
Classic clear pink

BROWN EYES
Wood rose

Redheads

Eyes

Veridian

Cinnamon

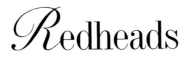

Soft charcoal

BLUE EYES
Camel

GREEN EYES
Golden brown

HAZEL EYES
Mocha

BROWN EYES
Teal

DARK BROWN EYES
Teal

Cheeks

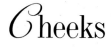

Beige matte blush

Cinnamon

BLUE EYES
Sandalwood

GREEN EYES
Pale mauve

HAZEL EYES
Tawny rouge

BROWN EYES
Silky mauve

DARK BROWN EYES
Bordeaux

Lips

Sienna

Cinnamon

BLUE EYES
Transparent bordeaux

GREEN EYES
Clear soft peach

HAZEL EYES
Gold copper

BROWN EYES
Peach bronze

DARK BROWN EYES
Bronze/Gold

Gray Hair

Eyes

Coffee

Nutmeg/Dark beige

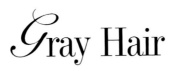

Mustard yellow

BLUE EYES
Gray mauve

GREEN EYES
Iris

HAZEL EYES
Willow green

BROWN EYES
Terra-cotta

DARK BROWN EYES
Viridian

*C*heeks   *L*ips

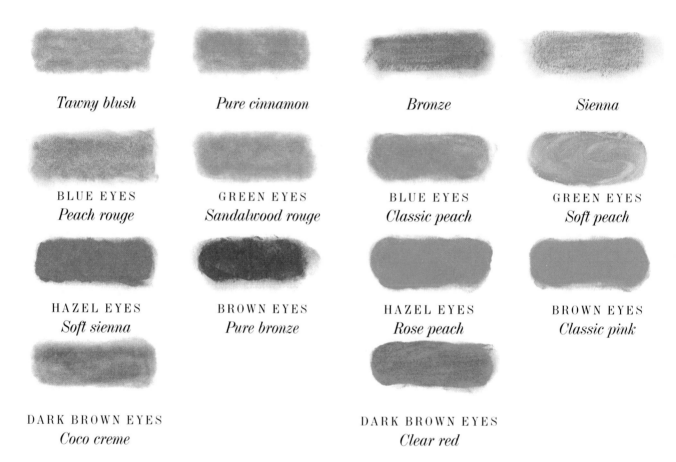

Cheeks		Lips	
Tawny blush	*Pure cinnamon*	*Bronze*	*Sienna*
BLUE EYES *Peach rouge*	GREEN EYES *Sandalwood rouge*	BLUE EYES *Classic peach*	GREEN EYES *Soft peach*
HAZEL EYES *Soft sienna*	BROWN EYES *Pure bronze*	HAZEL EYES *Rose peach*	BROWN EYES *Classic pink*
DARK BROWN EYES *Coco creme*		DARK BROWN EYES *Clear red*	

Exotics

Black Skin Eyes

Royal blue

Lavender

Mahogany

GREEN EYES
Granite

HAZEL EYES
Classic terra-cotta

LIGHT BROWN EYES
Charcoal

DARK BROWN EYES
Blue-gray

BROWN-BLACK EYES
Deep olive

Exotic Cheeks

Classic rose

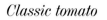

Classic tomato

Earth red

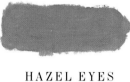

HAZEL EYES
Sienna

GREEN/GRAY
Classic mauve

LIGHT BROWN EYES
Mahogany

DARK BROWN EYES
Violet

BLACK EYES
Real mauve

Olive to Black Skin Lips

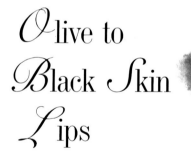

Bronze/Copper

Deep sienna orange

Matte red

HAZEL EYES
Burnt orange

GRAY-GREEN EYES
Clear mahogany

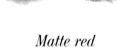

LIGHT BROWN EYES
Soft plum

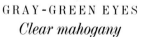

DARK BROWN EYES
Transparent red

DARK BROWN TO BLACK EYES
Classic red